The Mechanic and the Gardener

THE MECHANIC
and the
GARDENER

*Making the Most
of the Holistic
Revolution in
Medicine*

LAWRENCE
LeSHAN

HOLT, RINEHART AND WINSTON NEW YORK

Library of Congress Cataloging in Publication Data

LeShan, Lawrence L., 1920–
The Mechanic and the Gardener.
Includes bibliographical references.
1. Medicine—Philosophy.   2. Health.
3. Holistic medicine.   4. Medical personnel
and patient.   5. Self-care, Health.   I. Title.
R723.L47   613   81-19236
                AACR2

ISBN 0-03-059517-7

First Edition

Designer: Joy Chu
Printed in the United States of America
10 9 8 7 6 5 4 3 2 1

Grateful acknowledgment is made for use of quotations
from the following:
Patients and Doctors by Kenneth Walker,
copyright © 1957 by Kenneth Walker.
Reprinted by permission of Penguin Books Ltd.
The Case for Unorthodox Medicine by Brian Inglis,
copyright © 1967 by Brian Inglis.
Reprinted by permission of Curtis Brown Ltd.

ISBN 0-03-059517-7

TO ANNE APPELBAUM
with love and gratitude
who is responsible for many
of the ideas in this book and
has the most refreshing approach
to the field of medicine I have
ever known.

Contents

The Mechanic and the Gardener

Introduction

As a nation we spend over $250 billion a year on medical care. (Over $6 billion worth of prescriptions are written each year.) It is difficult to comprehend such figures—but one thing seems quite clear: most people don't feel it is enough. Patients complain that there are not enough doctors and nurses; doctors and nurses complain they don't have enough technicians, enough space, enough equipment. Hospitals get bigger and bigger—to such a point that it has become impossible to find one's way to a specific service without streaks of different colors along the floors or walls, and a map more complicated than those for most cross-country highways.

As in so many other spheres of life, the human need for personal attention, loving care, intimate contact hasn't changed, but everything has changed about medical services, so that while we hear daily about wonderful, thrilling new breakthroughs, medical discoveries that can save lives, most of us who need to have contact with doctors and hospitals usually feel lost, alone, confused, and anonymous. We lose our identity, we begin to feel we are nonpersons.

At the same time that it is surely true that more people are living longer due to the advances of modern medical knowledge and technology, we are also hearing horror stories about people who suffer desperately from new treatment methods, and people who receive wrong diagnoses, wrong treatments, whose records are lost, who are told ten different "truths" by ten different experts.

Frequently these different opinions leave the patient in the desperate situation of having to make life-and-death choices between therapy programs and having to do it on the basis of inadequate and conflicting information.

Every week we read about new medical discoveries and marvelous new techniques and we also know people with severe illnesses about which modern medicine seems unable to do anything constructive. In spite of very large amounts of research money spent on cancer, those with the disease seem to find that orthodox medicine has little to offer except harsher and harsher poisons used on the theory that they will kill the cancer cells before they finally kill the person, and more and more extensive surgery. The devastation caused by modern cancer chemotherapy and surgery is becoming a byword.

One of the most devastating features of the advances in medical techniques and knowledge has been the tendency to identify people by disease or by organ only. There is the classic story of the surgeon who tells his office nurse, "Send in the stomach case now, I'll see the liver after that." The more we learn about the *technical craft* of saving physical life, the less we seem to have kept in touch with the *human art* of caring about the person.

Recently I visited a hospital in West Virginia where I worked thirty-eight years ago. At that time it was a 2,500-bed army medical facility constantly full of the casualties of World War II. It was a one-story building and every ward faced the open air and had grass and trees on three sides. In spite of its size it was a close-knit and caring place with a warm and friendly atmosphere. Everyone, patients and staff alike, gathered in off-hours at the central recreation area, "Times Square," with its coffee shop, lounge areas, auditorium, and movies.

When I came back to it this year the place was still much the same. Now a veterans' hospital, it still retained in its wards and corridors the same warm, informal, and caring atmosphere it had had in the past. The countryside was still green all around it. The patient population tended to be older, but outside of that I couldn't find too much change. I talked informally to patients and staff and received the same impression from both. It is still a hospital where, if you are a patient, you know that the staff is primarily interested in taking care of you. You feel safe and protected.

A quarter of a mile behind it a new structure is being built. This is the new hospital that in a year or so will replace the old one. It is sixteen stories high, very modern; a giant box of a place. It will be technologically more efficient than the old rambling building. However, none of the wards will have open air on three sides nor will a patient be able to get out of bed, walk ten feet, and sit on a lawn. I know from experience that the entire atmosphere and tone of the place will also change. Concern will shift from patient care to technology. Patients will be less and less the central focus of the organization and more and more business criteria and engineering concepts will take their place. The rate of patient recovery will go down. In spite of the fact that every study has shown that recovery from serious illness takes place most rapidly in an intimate and caring environment, hospitals keep getting bigger and bigger and more oriented toward modern technology. The new building will probably save some money per patient day in the long run. It will also increase the average time patients stay and will thus have a higher cost in every way when the total picture is in.

In recent years—due in good part to the lack of caring for the whole person in mainline medicine—we have seen the remarkable and rapid rise of a new medical model, which generally is described as "holistic medicine." The term has come to mean a variety of things—from nutrition to acupuncture to psychic healing—but what all holistic methods have in common is the underlying hunger, the profound search, for some way to see and respond to the patient as a complete person, not just as a collection of functioning or nonfunctioning organs.

For what we are more and more aware of is that though the technology of medicine, the bigger and bigger hospitals, and the growing depersonalization thereby created may "fix up" a broken or diseased body, a return to health demands that the patient participate in the healing process, or it doesn't work.

The present public interest in "holistic medicine" in all forms, both sensible and silly, involving both practitioners of integrity and charlatans, has developed primarily because of this awareness that technology is not enough. The exact meaning of the term, however, eludes us. New modalities of treatment constantly appear, leaving us hopeful but confused.

A major part of the development, however, is clear. It is concerned with widening the view of the patient; with the understanding that *all* levels of his being are of equal importance in the prevention of disease and the search for health. In the cure of disease, this wider interest also has the purpose of bringing more strongly into play that patient's own self-healing and self-repair abilities—of bringing these capabilities to the aid of the medical program. These "other" levels comprise a wide range, from the nutritional to the spiritual, and include the patient's relationship needs and creative needs.

Approaches such as chiropractic, osteopathy, and homeopathy have existed side by side with the more traditional medical treatments for a very long time. New ways of seeking health are constantly appearing and being publicized. These range from acupuncture to meditation to new nutritional approaches to jogging to psychic healing to megavitamins and dozens of others.

Specialists in all these modalities are constantly exhorting us that they have *the* path toward health. Many of these approaches, both the new and the old, obviously have something of real value in them. But how shall a person judge? How shall a person take care of his own health amid such an overwhelming barrage of information and claims?

The purpose of this book is to try to give you the kind of information which will help you make such serious decisions; to give you a perspective on the field of medicine that will increase your awareness of alternatives. What has the past contributed to present attitudes and techniques? What is the present situation in all its ramifications? How can we make sound choices and judgments for ourselves and our families?

First of all I will try to describe the flood of medical information and misinformation that we are subjected to today in the newspapers and television. Why is this going on and what is it doing to us and to our attitudes about our own bodies? Although we tend to be somewhat aware of our own confusions, we are less likely to be aware of what this is doing to physicians, of the very heavy loads, both physically and psychologically, that are now placed on them. There is at present very little relationship between the physician's training and many of the tasks that are assigned to him. Both the lay public and the medical profession are, at this time, confused, angry, and disappointed.

There has been a conflict at the heart of medical practice since Roman times at least. This is the question as to whether the physician should concentrate on actively intervening in disease or whether his primary emphasis should be on helping the patient's self-healing systems to work more effectively. The viewpoints both of the public and the profession have swung back and forth on this question in different historical periods. It is this problem which is at the center of the present confusion about "holistic medicine." We are now reaching for a new synthesis of the two viewpoints, an understanding of the strengths and weaknesses of both. We are beginning to learn where each is useful and how best to combine them.

The revolution in science that has taken place in this century has profoundly affected our new concept of disease and health. The heart of this revolution is the idea that different ways of dealing with problems and different ways of thinking about them are necessary with different kinds of experience. We are beginning to understand that we need an approach to the problem of "health" different from that which we apply to the problem of "disease."

The problems of curing disease are different from the problems of searching for health. A large part of our confusion in the medical field has come about because we have confused these two and considered health the absence of disease. As we begin to see the differences between these two separate realms, we can approach them with the methods and viewpoints relevant to each.

Going even further, it seems clear to me that, in the future, we are going to need two separate kinds of specialists: specialists in disease and specialists in health. One will help us prevent and cure disease—the breakdown of our ability to function. The other will help us move toward health—the zest, gusto, and serenity of life that give us a *reason* for functioning, stimulate our self-repair and self-healing systems, and make us far less vulnerable to disease. These two kinds of specialists will need different kinds of personalities and types of training.

Probably the most important issue in this book is the challenge for each person to become his or her own health specialist. Since there is now very little selection or training of health specialists, and only a few of them exist, it will be necessary for some time yet for most people to function as their own. A method for exploring and fulfilling your own health needs will be described, and there will also be a discussion of the adjunctive modalities (such as nutrition, acupuncture, homeopathy) that are so much in the news these days. Suggestions will be made as to how to choose adjunctive modalities for your own use and how to evaluate the practitioners of these methods.

With the advances in size and available technology, the modern hospital has frequently become more oriented to profit making (from the sale of tests, procedures, and bed

space) than patient care. It is important that you (or someone close to you who can act as your advocate) know how
to obtain the most benefit, and have the least harm done,
by your hospital stay. A "survival kit" of both information
and objects will be suggested for hospital patients.

This book has been a long time in the writing; about forty years, as a matter of fact! As a young psychologist in the
1940s, I was led by my training to the belief that *I* knew all
about mental illness and mental health, and my patients
knew nothing—until, of course, I had passed my wisdom
on to them!

Something happened early in my career that helped me
to grow up—to begin to understand the inner strengths and
wisdom of all human beings. I began to work on a research
project that involved psychotherapy with cancer patients. I
quickly discovered that the nice, neat theories I'd been
taught about emotional pathology were almost useless
when I sat—as I did for thousands of hours—in my office
talking to men and women facing a catastrophic illness and
possible death. I learned that while the first half of being a
psychologist might, indeed, be to learn all one could about
human problems, the second half of one's training required
a growing awareness of all the qualities I had to recognize
among my patients—qualities like courage, sensitivity, compassion for others, a profound sense of morality, and most
of all, an inner wisdom about what they really needed in
life that could mobilize their resources and help them to
get well.

Many years after starting the cancer research project, I
became interested in the field of psychic phenomena—
what we call paranormal events. In the course of exploring
this area, I spent a number of years investigating psychic
healing, and once again I was to marvel at the remarkable
capacity human beings have for knowing what they need
and knowing what can help them to make themselves well.

It took many years of growth on my part to appreciate

fully the fact that while there, of course, are all kinds of advice and counsel and direct medical intervention that can be helpful to people, none of these professional skills can be of much use at all unless there is a profound respect for each person's own judgment of who he or she is and what is needed for the fullest healthy potential in living. It is with that appreciation of universal inner wisdom that I offer the guidelines discussed in this book.

THE PRESENT SITUATION
IN MEDICINE

That any sane nation, having observed that you could provide for the supply of bread by giving bakers a pecuniary interest in baking for you, should go on to give surgeons a pecuniary interest in cutting off your leg, is enough to make one despair of political humanity.

—GEORGE BERNARD SHAW

1

We are bombarded by the media with the message that "your health is a mess. To stave off disaster, you should immediately take a medication or see a professional." Lewis Thomas (president of New York's Memorial Sloan-Kettering Cancer Center) recently wrote:

> Nothing has changed so much in the past twenty-five years as the public's perception of its own health. The change amounts to a loss of confidence in the human form. The general belief these days [1977] seems to be that the body is fundamentally flawed, subject to disintegration at any moment, always on the verge of mortal disease, always in need of continual monitoring and support by health-care professionals.

> Our new view is close to that of many primitive societies, that death is unnatural; that it should not happen. The primitive says that a witch or a demon caused it. The modern says that the doctor failed to prevent it.

There is a tremendous amount of propaganda from drug companies and their advertising agencies to the effect that our bodies do not work and are constantly in danger of decomposing from one thing or another. We must, we are warned, keep a large variety of drugs available, or we will certainly be overcome with everything from dandruff through hemorrhoids to athlete's foot. Not a single system of the body (excluding those like the lymphatic that the lay public does not really believe exist) is exempted from the threat that it cannot function well by itself or recover unaided if it becomes disordered. We are further warned that there are really severe and terrible problems awaiting us and that we had better prepare for them by giving money to specialized foundations so that their research can be further advanced by the time their particular dread disease fells us or someone close to us. There is no effective counterpropaganda around. No agency exists for the celebration of the fact that most people are, in real life, free of active disease and will recover from any minor indisposition by themselves. "No one takes public note of the truth of the matter, which is that most people in this country have a clear, unimpeded run at a longer lifetime than could have been foreseen by an earlier generation."

Indeed one of the easiest ways of making people angry at you (try it on your friends and watch them become your former friends) is to tell them that they do *not* need more medical care, vitamins, exercise, dietary expertise, or constant concern about their health. This has become the equivalent of a personal attack in most circles and will generally elicit the same response you would get if you were to light a cigarette in a health-foods store.

In spite of the fact that the amount spent in this country on medical care rose from $10 billion in 1950 to $250 billion in 1980, we all feel that the medical system is underfinanced and inadequate, that physicians are too hurried and overworked, and that there are not enough nurses. Further, if you examine medical progress, there should logically have been a lowering of health costs.

A typical case of lobar pneumonia, pre-antibiotic, involved three or four weeks of hospitalization; typhoid was a twelve-to-sixteen week illness; meningitis often required several months of care through convalescence; these and other common infectious diseases can now be aborted promptly, within just a few days. The net result of the anti-infection technology ought to have been a very large decrease in the cost of care.

We feel angry when we are told that we have long since reached a point of diminishing returns in pumping more money into the medical system; that we are, as a nation, remarkably free of disease and far more so than at any other period; that our bodies are generally capable of taking care of themselves; and that we should stop feeling guilty that we are not taking better care of our physical being. Hearing these things, we feel as if we are being attacked and something is being taken away from us.

And, indeed, something *is* being taken away. It is the hope of magic: the hope that medicine (with its magicians dressed in white coats) will solve all our problems; postpone death until we are ready—or, perhaps, forever—and make us "healthy," and full of zest, joy, and sexual attractiveness and ability. Anyone who takes away the hope that we can achieve heaven on earth if we only take a few more milligrams of vitamin C *plus* zinc *plus* vitamin E each day is going to be cordially disliked. Our belief in the magical promise of medicine is an illusion of our entire culture today, and anyone who tries to remove that belief does so at his peril.

However, there is a reason to try to give up this illusion, and to point out its fallacy. The illusion leads to a blocking of our perceptions, so that we cannot see how we can validly work toward our own health. It leads to the placement of tremendous and unfair loads on the medical profession, and to a continuing and increasing hostility between the physician and the lay public as medical capabilities do not live up to the impossible hopes we have for them. It is also turning us into a nation of angry and overmedicated hypochondriacs.

Paradoxically, we are as a culture extremely discontented with the entire medical system. An HEW study reported that in 1979 only 7 percent of Americans identified themselves as "feeling good most of the time." How did we get into this predicament?

There are, I believe, three major ways to account for it:

1. The rise of the mechanical view in Western society and the concomitant idea that *everything* can be fixed and made to run perfectly.
2. The tremendous advances of medicine in the last century. Control of the communicable and infectious diseases led to the idea that *all* diseases could be controlled.
3. The confusion that identified health as "an absence of disease." This semantic disaster led us to the idea we would be "healthy" when free of disease.

Since we all knew we wanted something called "health" very badly, but had not defined it, and since we knew that it was something we could get by curing "sickness," an entire industry grew up to try to satisfy this need. Working on the principle that if what you are doing doesn't work, do it more—if the bolt does not fit the nut, force it until it does— medical procedures grew more and more extensive. The use of surgery, drugs, yearly medical examinations, tonics, vitamins, and so forth increased exponentially. As with any competitive industry, the means often replaced the end, and what could be sold became as much a hallmark of

validity as did the products' effectiveness. Many of the procedures and products were useless (such as yearly examinations and wholesale tonsil removal) and some were
downright dangerous (the thalidomide and DES disasters
are only the tip of the iceberg now emerging).

A part of our present problem is a linguistic one. We
tend to speak of a disease as a "thing," and not as part of a
total life process. We thereby separate the person and the
illness. This automatically leads us back to the old demon
theory of disease in which a demon invaded the body and
had to be dispossessed. As soon as the demon was driven
out, the person was cured. It would be far more realistic, in
terms of modern knowledge (and would improve our ability to solve problems in this area), to restructure our language so that when we spoke or thought about illness, the
language would indicate that the specific individual had tensions, strengths, and weaknesses in his relationship with
himself, others, and the cosmos, and that this total gestalt
was showing symptoms of carcinoma or of angina pectoris.
We would then automatically see any healing process as
having two interrelated parts: emergency treatment of the
symptom and long-term reorganization of the total pattern
of the person's life.

Because we see the disease and the illness as a "thing"
that has happened to us, we seek a "cause." The use of
"fate" or "happenstance" to explain untoward events is no
more acceptable in our society than is the evil eye of a bad-
tempered witch doctor. We may, for example, lay the blame
on "carcinogens" in the air, forgetting that while these *are* a
real threat to our defense systems, they do not affect in the
same way all persons equally exposed. Nevertheless, it is
useful and soothing to have an acceptable demon out there
and to attempt—as we should and must—to clean up our
air and water. It *is* important that we do this, but if we believe that these outside factors are the sole cause of illness,
we are going to be disappointed and depressed if we even-

tually do have air that is fit for us and our children to breathe and disease continues. The environment is only one factor in the pattern, not the sole "cause" of illness.

We often try to blame other people—"My boss caused the heart attack by being such a bastard"—although unless we have a sizable paranoid streak in our personality make-up, this kind of explanation doesn't feel very satisfying for very long. Since Freud, a new explanation has become popular in our culture. "In our society psychosomatic explanations of illness have become extremely popular because they allow patients to fix the blame on the most comforting locus of all—themselves."

The idea that there is a single cause for illness, that something or someone must be to blame, can often be heard in the sound of a patient's voice as he asks his physician: "Why have I contracted this disease?" The tone implies that something underhanded is going on. We want there to be a simple cause, preferably something outside of ourselves, and to know that we contracted the disease by chance. The answer "A virus" and the assurance that "there's a lot of it going around" fits our wishes exactly. We can neglect to ask why others similarly exposed did not also contract the disease. We want the doctor to be able to repel the invader with no particular inconvenience to ourselves (except perhaps for a shot, a pill, and a few days in bed) and with no implication that the illness may be telling us something about taking on further responsibility for our own lives.

The idea of one specific cause for each disease, and therefore, one specific cure, fits in well with another of our fantasies.

There is a very old belief among human beings that somewhere there exists a "natural" remedy, a plant or herb, that will solve all human medical problems and give us health and youth forever—in short, that it will make us immortal. This belief goes back at least to Sumerian times. We find it in the Gilgamesh saga probably composed before 3000 B.C. The surgeon and philosopher Kenneth Walker believes that this belief comes in part from observations of the behavior of animals, who will often treat themselves for wounds or illness by eating certain plants or by using material in their natural environment. Birds, for example, are very successful in ridding themselves of insect parasites by means of dust baths. (It is only recently that we have understood that this works by clogging up the respiratory pores of the insects.) The belief is very persistent, and finds its modern equivalent today in many of the kooky fad diets and advertisements for over-the-counter remedies that clutter up the media. So deeply ingrained is this idea in Western culture that one nineteenth-century German medical research scientist felt it necessary to try to disabuse his students and associates of it by putting a plaque over the entrance of his laboratory: *"Gegen den Todt ist keine Kraut gewachsen."* (Against death do no herbs grow.)

The widespread fantasy of a Golden Age that preceded our own (whatever our own might be) has also confounded the present concept of sickness and health. We have a feeling that in a previous age human beings were happier and healthier than they are now. If we stop to think about it, we quickly realize that this is not so, but the notion persists and influences our viewpoint to a very marked degree. We feel, for example, that in the small town of sixty years ago (a sort of cross between Andy Hardy's hometown and a stage set for Thornton Wilder's *Our Town*) with its good and caring physician (probably looking a bit like Lionel Barrymore) there was less sickness. Thus, the nutritionists blame most of today's illness on chemical additives in our food, and the American Cancer Society blames most cancers on environmental carcinogens produced by the industry of our time. Both of these theories seem reasonable until we look at the mortality statistics of the past century and it becomes clear that these explanations are too simplistic.

As one example, I might mention that in Egyptian mummies (from the best families of Egypt and long before environmental poisons and food additives) we find ample evidence of widespread tumors, arthritis, caries, silicosis, pneumonia, pleurisy, rheumatism, kidney stones, cirrhosis of the liver, mastoiditis, appendicitis, meningitis, smallpox, TB, and a wide variety of other conditions.

The idea of a golden age of health preceding ours is not a new one. In 1796, the physician C. W. Hufeland wrote that mankind was on the road to physical degeneration and a higher early death rate, unless it returned to the simple ways of life of the good old times "in ways agreeable to nature."

Since Rousseau in particular, and the French Revolution in general, the idea has been prevalent that it is society that causes illnesses, and that in a "natural state" (whatever that means) or in a "good society" (defined by the beliefs of the moment), people would be healthy and not have disease. (The latest version of this notion is the rapidly growing belief that *everything* produced by modern technology is carcinogenic.) The belief is that once the revolution (the changes *we* advocate) is complete, people will be free of disease. Excuses when this does not happen are as ingenious and plentiful among revolutionists as they are among Christian Scientists.

It must be made clear that what is being said in this chapter is not a criticism of physicians, but an analysis of the present-day structure of medicine and its position in our society. The physician is generally in practice for serious and positive motives, and is under more pressure from medicine's structure and status than is the layman.

In the 1940s, the World Health Organization defined *health* as "a state of complete physical, mental, and social well-being." This definition places a tremendous burden on those who are expected to deal with health problems: the members of the medical profession. They are rather well equipped to deal with the first third of the definition (physical), ill equipped to deal with the second (mental), and completely unequipped to deal with the third (social). Neither were they trained to deal with the constant interaction among the three, nor to recognize that the definition omits a crucial part of what it means to be human—the spiritual, the deep and basic need to have a meaningful framework for existence. Forgotten was the obvious fact, shown throughout history, that human beings will often sacrifice their physical well-being in order to satisfy their spiritual needs.

It is part of the swing of the cultural pendulum that today the welfare of a population is considered almost entirely in secular terms. In the reaction to the medieval view that the welfare of the soul was of primary importance, we have, since the eighteenth century, been moving in the opposite direction, toward the view that the welfare of the body is of sole importance. This is one reason we have been concerned with "sickness" (something wrong with the body) rather than "health" (something right with the entire organism). The months of meetings of the council of the French Revolution on how best to replace the clergy with a medical bureaucracy was a very clear example of this development, which we are only now beginning seriously to challenge.

Since "health" was seen merely as the absence of "sickness," increasingly the problems associated with being human tended to become included in the definition of illness. During the past sixty years the physician has been constantly assigned more and more tasks—many of which he has had no training in handling. The lack of "happiness," "fulfillment," and "zest in life" has been defined as illness. This has gradually become part of the physician's responsibility, a problem that he is expected to be able to "cure." None of these, of course, are problems that machines have and so are out of the range of the basic system around which medical training is organized.

So great has been the medicalization of American society, to use an expression of the biometrician Renée Fox, that the hospital is succeeding the church or the parliament as the archetypical institution of Western society. Disapproved behavior is coming to be considered illness requiring treatment rather than crime requiring punishment or sin requiring conversion.

Anything that the physician is willing to deal with becomes an illness and the implication is reinforced that only physicians are able to deal with it or that they are more effective with the problem than anyone else. Thus the physician says that he is willing to treat alcoholism, since it is a negative deviation from a norm and that is how he defines a disease. Alcoholism thus *becomes* a disease, and the physician's prerogative to treat, even though he does not know the cause and has no reason to suspect that the cause is biological. Further, there is no reason to suspect that he is more effective dealing with it than are the courts or the church, and he is less successful than the peer treatment of A.A.

Medicalization has gone so far that we no longer even believe in our ability to die alone or in the warmth of the company of our loved ones. We feel that we must have around us a court of white-coated antiseptic figures to make the final transition. The individual has come to feel so helpless that he cannot even wrestle with his own death or find his own path to it.

Before the beginning of this century, the modern physician's case load was divided between two classes of professionals. A large part of his present practice went to the health professionals of that era—the religious. (Or to the "wise" advisors of the community.) Problems that they once handled, and which now come to the consulting room, include: addictive disorders such as alcoholism, drug abuse, and obesity, the "worried well," who make up such a large part of the physician's everyday medical work, certain types of physical violence such as that leading to the

"battered child" or "battered wife" syndrome, existential crises, inability to conceive or to stop conceiving, discontent
with a job or love life, bedwetting, sexual deviance and dysfunction, anorexia nervosa, mental or physical exhaustion,
difficulty in relating to others, inability to find meaning in
life, and unhappiness. Even pregnancy is—in practice—generally regarded as a nine-month self-limiting illness, often
requiring surgery at the end. In the Soviet Union, dis-
agreement with the dictates of the Central Committee is seen
as prima facie evidence of mental illness, and the political
dissident is likely to become a medical "patient" and wind
up in a mental hospital.

In Maoist China, mental illness was perceived as a political problem and Maoist politicians were placed in charge of
psychotic deviants. (It is not clear if this has recently
changed.) The psychotic was perceived as a person who
was—at least unconsciously—a class enemy who needed
criticism and self-criticism to make him politically active and
therefore healthy.

In the United States we do the same thing, but generally
limit the punishment to children who have no votes. Those
children who object to poor teaching and poor educational
theory are turned over to the medical arm of the establish-
ment for drugging and retraining. The belief is that drugs
like Ritalin will cure them of their objections to an educational system on the brink of disaster. (We also do occasionally use medical definitions for political purposes. Two
cases in this category would be those of Ezra Pound and
General James Walker.)

As for the use of drugs for "hyperactive" children (that
is to say, children who aren't school adjusted), our present
approach is also used by at least one primitive culture.
Among the Jivaro Indians of South America (one of the
most hostile and aggressive societies ever discovered) if a
child consistently misbehaves he is forcibly administered a
very powerful hallucinogen (datura). The theory is that this

will enable him to perceive "reality" correctly, and he will then start to behave. How this approach differs from our own (except in the choice of drug used) escapes my understanding.

Further, the physician must now decide who may drive a car, stay away from work, immigrate, become a soldier; who is competent to know right from wrong, or is likely to be dangerous to himself or others, or is too hopelessly ill to be worthy of further use of life-saving devices; who is too incompetent to manage his own affairs; who receives the first available organ for transplant, and who must wait. With this kind of assignment and the kind of training they get, is it any wonder that physicians have such high heart-attack, drug-abuse, and suicide rates? (Suicide is the second most common cause of death for medical students and is more frequent among physicians than the combined deaths from automobile accidents, airplane crashes, homicides, and drownings. Drugs and alcohol account for at least one-third of the time physicians as a group spend hospitalized during their careers.)

With the medicalization of American society, the physician now has the power to legitimize one's "illness" (the feeling of being sick) by conceding that one actually has a disease. He also has the power to deny this legitimacy. If you are not ill in the correct ways with the correct symptoms, you are labeled a hypochondriac, a malingerer (if you seem to be gaining a financial advantage), or a neurotic. The penalties for being sick in incorrect ways can range from social ostracism to denial of workmen's compensation funds. The penalties for being sick in incorrect ways in the army or in prison are obvious.

Some years ago, a patient came to me for psychotherapy. Her major symptom was that she became sick every time she ate in a Chinese restaurant. No such reaction was then recognized in medical circles, and several medical specialists she had seen had suggested psychotherapy. After a

bit of exploring it seemed clear that her major symptom indeed was that she became sick after eating in Chinese restaurants. I recommended that she stop eating in them. She
followed this brilliant recommendation and stopped being
ill. Several years later it became known to physicians (and
was reported in the best journals) that some people had a
negative reaction to monosodium glutamate, which is extensively used in Chinese restaurants. The patient now had
a disease with a label and was advised by her doctor not to
eat in Chinese restaurants.

This may seem a rather minor and humorous case (although not to the woman involved), but the matter can be
far more serious. If your illness or your disease does not fit
the textbook requirements, or if you do not respond to
medical intervention in the way that physicians think that
you should, the physician may not only label you a hysteric,
he may simply want nothing more to do with you and treat
you in a superficial "don't bother me, I'm busy" manner. He
may resort to more and more assaultive treatments, or may
simply get rid of you completely, as you are disturbing to
his peace of mind. By not responding in the approved and
standardized way, you threaten to make the physician think
about you as an individual and to relate to you as a total
person, not just as a disease or a broken machine. As he has
not been trained to do this, and—indeed—has been trained
to do the opposite, this can be very upsetting to him.

In the late 1970s, I knew a man who was in New York's
famed Memorial Hospital with a metastasized prostate cancer. He had had surgery and chemotherapy, which had
failed to stop the spread of the cancer. The oncologist in
charge of the case then strongly urged him to undergo a
surgical castration, to which he agreed. One week later, still
in severe pain from the operation, he was told that it had
not worked, that the hospital had nothing more to offer
him, and that he would have to leave immediately in order
to make room for patients who could be successfully treat-

ed. He was then forced to leave the hospital before he could find another that would admit him. After several days at home, in great pain, he was admitted to another hospital, at which he died.

The nineteenth-century definition of medicine, which medical schools are still using, was "The science concerned with the prevention and cure of disease." The authoritative *Stedman's Medical Dictionary* defines disease as: "Morbus, Illness, Sickness. An interruption or perversion of functions of any of the organs, a morbid change in any of the tissues or an abnormal state of the body as a whole, continuing for a longer or shorter period." This is what the physician has been trained to cope with and essentially all the physician has been trained to cope with.

In every profession, a certain amount of "ethnocentrism" develops. (George Bernard Shaw wrote, "Every profession is a conspiracy against the layman.") The lawyer sacrifices the larger view of humanity for a concentration on property and torts, the cleric on sanctity, the academician on learning, the chef on eating, and the physician on illness and therapy. The population is seen from a specialized point of view, and actions are inevitably interpreted in the light of this view rather than from a more universal perspective.

Trained to look for sickness, very often the physician can *see* only sickness and cannot perceive normal functioning. Individual variations in function and in behavior are much too easily perceived as pathology. In one experiment eight pseudo patients had themselves admitted to mental institutions by saying that they heard voices. Thereafter they behaved normally. The entire staff remained convinced that they were "schizophrenics" as labeled, and did not recognize their lack of psychosis. The staff did not seem capable of recognizing normal behavior in patients, although some of the other patients suspected the impersonations. An experiment with highly trained psychoanalysts produced much the same results.

Thomas Szasz has pointed out that if a psychiatrist refers a patient for personality testing, the presumption is that the patient is ill and, consequently, the psychologist finds psychopathology.

In more than twenty years of psychiatric work, I have never known a clinical psychologist to report, on the basis of a projective test, that the subject is a "normal, mentally healthy person." While some witches may have survived dunking and been acquitted by the water test as innocent, no "modern" survives psychological testing.

One factor making progress in medicine more difficult has been the belief, in our era, in simplification. This is the idea that as we understand more about something, its structure becomes more obvious and simple and our explanations become less complex. Ultimately, we have believed, one unified field theory would explain everything in the cosmos. In medicine, this has tended to mean that we expect ultimately to find one cause for each disease, a specific bacterium for this, a specific virus for that. In pursuing this concept, we have left out the tremendous differences among our patients, the fact that each sick person is an entire universe with positive and negative forces interacting in very intricate ways. The idea that increased knowledge brings simplification is deeply rooted in our culture. As the current revolution in physics has shown, however, sometimes as we come to know more, we find that things are increasingly complicated. With our increased knowledge of quantum mechanics and relativity theory, physics has certainly not become more simple but more complex.

Another factor leading to the increase in the physician's psychological load has been an assumption that has gradually developed in our culture during the last century. This is the idea that no matter what the problem, there is a trained technologist or scientist who can solve it; that someone else (or a mechanical technique of some kind) will solve the problem for you. As machines became more and more efficient, the belief developed that they—or their substitutes, such as pills—could do anything. We learned to depend less and less on ourselves and our own hard work, our own self-development, and our own self-healing abilities. In medicine, the physician was expected to have a "magic bullet" for all problems including our unease at the state of our lives and our unhappiness at our lack of self-fulfillment. It was inevitable that a drug culture and a medicalized society would develop from this assumption.

The medicalization of Western society has proceeded with great rapidity. What has resulted is a greater and greater dependency on medicine and an increasing anger at the profession for failing to succeed completely, for failing to provide us with that undefined entity—health. (The present tendency to sue for malpractice at the slightest opportunity is only one symptom of this anger.)

Under the threat to physicians of increased numbers of malpractice suits, we seem bent on returning to the medical situation of ancient Egypt. There the physician was forced—under the threat of severe punishment—to treat a disease by the officially prescribed method and that alone. The difference is that the Egyptians were less rigid than we are in danger of becoming. After four days, if there was no improvement, the Egyptian physician was allowed to use his creativity and try other methods.

A further interesting similarity is shown in the degree of specialization common to ancient Egyptian and contemporary physicians. Since the body was believed by the ancient Egyptians to have thirty-six parts, they had thirty-six kinds of specialists. Today we have thirty-six Board-certified specialties. (I must add that this parallel is due to coincidence. There is no relationship between the thirty-six parts of the body the Egyptians conceived of and thirty-six modern-day Board specialties.)

There is even a strain of Utopian thinking that says: If people were "healthy," they would not fight wars. Whatever the ultimate truth of this idea, so long as health is defined only as the absence of disease, it is not very helpful. No one has yet demonstrated a relationship between sanitation procedures and peacefulness. Medical practices in the first half of this century in Switzerland and Germany were about the same: military adventurism was not.

Because our definition of "health" is so unclear, we are never satisfied. We keep believing that more money, physicians, clinics, and so forth will solve the problem. But we spent $10 billion for health in 1950 and $250 billion in 1980 and we seem as far as ever from our goal. It seems clear that something is very wrong with our method of searching for health. There is the old story of a man who saw, one night, a friend on his hands and knees, crawling around the base of a lamppost. On being asked why, the friend responded that he had lost the keys to his house and was searching for them. The man joined his friend in the search and after a few minutes with no success asked if he were sure he had lost them here. "Oh, no," replied the friend, "I lost them in the alley across the street, but there's more light to look by over here."

This is very similar to the present situation in medicine. We are looking for "health" in the wrong place—as an absence of disease—and so no matter how hard we look or how much money we invest, we are not going to find it.

In the terms of the general attitude that has developed that health is an absence of sickness, and that the physician must take the active role and "do something" about each problem, the physician and the patient have painted themselves into a very difficult corner. The task of the physician is to "fix" the problem and the responsibility is seen as his, not the patient's. When we go to a physician with a problem, we have very much the same attitude that we have when we bring our car to a mechanic. "It's slow to start in the morning," we say. "Please fix it." We expect the mechanic to do something physically, not to tell the car that it must change its attitude, its owner, or that it is an Oldsmobile and has been living its life as if it were a Buick just because Buicks were the admired cars this year. We do not expect the mechanic to tell us that the car has the ability to fix itself and that we have to find out what is blocking this ability. If he cannot fix the car, we call him an incompetent and find another mechanic who will.

When we approach a physician in the same way—and, being a creature of the same culture, the physician has the same attitudes and expectations that we have—we force him to "do something" about the problem. The result is that the patient generally leaves the office medicated, frequently overmedicated, sometimes with completely unnecessary surgical procedures scheduled. And all because we regard ourselves as a machine to be fixed rather than an organism to be gardened.

A gardener has quite a different attitude. If something is wrong with the development of a plant, the gardener will examine the total environment in which the plant exists and to which it is responding. How do its genetically determined needs and potentialities interact with the environment? (In human beings we call this interaction the "life-style.") The gardener will then determine what the plant needs—more or less sun, minerals, acid-base balance in its nourishment, space around it, and so on. (To continue the analogy to humans, which of its physical, mental, interpersonal, or spiritual needs are under, over, or wrongly fed?) The gardener deals with the whole—with the organism in an environment. The mechanic fixes nonfunctioning parts. This is why it seems plain that for human "sickness" and "health," two different attitudes are needed. Although some wise professionals may be able to encompass both, it seems clear that for the foreseeable future we are going to need two separate sets of professionals working together.

A machine is "sick" when it is not functioning efficiently and needs a mechanic to fix it. It is "healthy" when it is running smoothly and does not need a mechanic. Similarly, in spite of all the definitions and arguments, Western culture defines a human being as sick when he needs a physician and healthy when he does not. *The definition of health used today is the absence of sickness.* When you analyze all the modern talk about "health-care delivery systems," you find that these words simply mean systems for connecting an individual the culture defines as sick to a medical practitioner. In fact, there are no such things as "health-care delivery systems," there are only connection systems for sick people and physicians.

That the present-day medical view of humans is the same as that of mechanics toward machines can be shown in a wide variety of examples. One would be that "underachieving" is seen as a problem to be "fixed," while "overachieving" is not. A machine needs fixing when it is not efficient enough, not when it is too efficient.

However, every gardener and every farmer knows that this is not true of living organisms. For a plant to grow beyond its optimum growth rate or beyond its optimum size is a sign of real trouble and breakdown. Overachievement in a plant is seen as a problem. In a machine or a human, it is not.

When a physician, viewing a patient's aging body as a rapidly wearing-out machine, says—or agrees with the patient's statement—that a symptom is due to aging, or when he says something idiotic like "What can you expect at your age? You know you're not a spring chicken anymore," he is reinforcing the patient's sense of helplessness at an inexorable loss of control, of impotence and gradual dissolution in the face of an inexorable process. This reinforcement of helplessness weakens the patient's ability to fight for control of his life. If you told an artist that his paintings would eventually decay and be lost, you would be telling him a truth. You certainly would not be helping the development of his creativity.

A meaningful answer would be, "Let us see what we can

do to lessen the effect of the symptom, if we cannot erase it completely, and let us go on to see in what ways the entire fabric of your life can be enhanced and made more rich and colorful." An answer of this sort reinforces the patient's sense of himself as a human being and aids him in taking control of his own destiny.

The physician will frequently say to the patient something like "A lot depends on your attitude." What is generally meant by this is: "If you are a good patient and do as I say and do not ask uncomfortable questions, it will be a lot easier on me and I will not have to deal with you as a human being who is suffering." One patient with a severe cancer observed that his physicians all spoke about his attitude and how important it was, but became extremely uncomfortable and changed the subject when he or his family mentioned activities like prayer, support groups, psychic healing, meditation, or psychotherapy—all things you do to change your attitude. Since machines do not have attitudes, the patient's physicians simply did not know how to respond to this kind of procedure. By and large, physicians who advocate positive attitudes are unhappy with any discussion of techniques to attain them, except the most superficial approaches. Thus, Carl Simonton—who prescribes meditation for his cancer patients as well as mainline medical techniques (he is a Board-certified Radiologist)—is often discounted by other cancer physicians because his methods go against their basic assumptions that they are dealing with the problems of a machine and that there is something queer and upsetting in dealing with a machine's mind. The same thing is true of the attitude of many physicians to their psychiatric colleagues. They feel that as soon as the psychiatrist does anything but administer drugs, he is departing from "real medicine," that he has left the province of science (which they see as the nineteenth-century mechanistic model of physics) and is trafficking in softheaded irrelevancies. (The development in many hospitals today of

"Liaison Psychiatrists"—psychiatrists who are assigned to other medical departments than psychiatry and who offer their special skills where needed in these departments—is beginning to change this picture.)

Another aspect of the problem is a conviction—held by physicians and patients alike—that doctors treat diseases. In truth, doctors treat people who have diseases. Forgetting this, doctors forget the people. It is the task of the health specialist to remember this, and, in remembering, to help the patient remember the meaning of his own existence.

A patient is a person with a disease (a dysfunction of processes), an illness (how he feels), and a life-style. All three come together in a pattern before he visits the doctor's office. They can no longer be usefully and meaningfully separated. If they are separated, we do violence to the integrity of the person and thereby contribute to the obstacles that impede his recovery. This is not to say that we cannot choose where to put our primary efforts. It may be necessary first to concentrate on controlling the infection, bandaging the wound, mobilizing the person to start changing his or her nutrition and exercise pattern, or to examine the quality of the person's life. However, unless we are clear that the disease, the illness, and the life-style are all part of the pattern, we either will not know where to commence or will forget to finish a course of treatment.

> The present trend of medicine is toward artificial health, toward a kind of directed physiology. . . . We still consider a human being to be a poorly constructed machine, whose parts must constantly be reinforced or repaired. . . . Artificial health does not suffice for human happiness. . . . The growing dissatisfaction of the public with the medical profession is, in some measure, due to the existence of this evil. We must help . . . [the] whole perform its functions efficiently rather than intervene ourselves in the work of each organ.

Instead of resembling a machine produced in series, man should, on the contrary, emphasize his uniqueness. In order to reconstruct personality, we must break the frame of the school, factory and office, and reject the very principles of technological civilization.

This concept has led, at times, to the development of what we might call "assaultive therapies." If a machine stops functioning, you inject something into it (such as oil or fuel) or find the broken part and remove it. Or else you simply throw the entire machine on the scrap pile, as we do by throwing people into mental hospitals or turning them loose so stiff and rigid with overdoses of Thorazine or Haldol that they can barely function. Anyone who has seen the inhabitants of a geriatric center paralyzed with Thorazine will know the truth of this. (Both of these, of course, are extremely useful drugs if used correctly.)

Every experienced physician knows what a deadly symptom has appeared when a patient with a serious disease says, "I just don't care about getting better. Life doesn't mean very much to me." Or other statements of this sort. Conversely, the physician also knows of the importance of the will to live, and the significance of the general patterns of life in determining the outcome of disease. In addition, he has seen how often premature retirement leads to decline and death, and how infants who are not held and loved enough die at a much higher rate from all causes than do infants not so deprived. However, because of the physician's mechanistic training and viewpoint, and because he basically sees himself—and is seen by his patients—as a repairman, he tends to become extremely uncomfortable in the presence of approaches that *do something* about these factors. Psychiatry is seen as inferior to "real" medicine; meditation and prayer as superstitions at worst or weak occupational therapy at best. The physician tends to ignore the implications of a proved and major symptom because it does not fit in with his system of thought. Physicians, as do other people, sometimes subscribe to the maxim "If the fact disagrees with your theory, put the fact under the rug and out of sight."

George Engel, one of the world's leading specialists and pioneers in psychosomatic medicine, wrote:

> The dominant model of diseases today is biomedical, with molecular biology its basic scientific discipline. It assumes disease to be fully accounted for by deviations from the norm of measurable biological (somatic) variables. It leaves no room within its framework for the social, psychological, and behavioral dimensions of illness. The biomedical model not only requires that disease be dealt with as an entity independent of social behavior, it also demands that behavioral aberrations be explained on the basis of disordered somatic (biochemical or neurophysiological) processes. Thus the biomedical model embraces both reductionism, the philosophic view that complex phenomena are ultimately derived from a single primary principle, and mind-body dualism, the doctrine that separates the mental from the somatic.

Engel goes on to say that the biomedical model is also the folk or popular model of medicine and influences future physicians long before they start their training. The training then, of course, reinforces it. "The biomedical model has thus become a cultural imperative, its limitations easily overlooked. In brief, it has now acquired the status of *dogma*."

Engel proceeds to point out that the complaints of patients (and the general feeling in Western society) that their health needs are not being met, are not only due to "unrealistic expectations," as many physicians have argued. They also reflect ". . . a genuine discrepancy between illness as actually experienced by the patient and as it is conceptualized in the biomedical mode." The patient is *ill* and needs healing. The physician sees a *disease* that needs *curing* and acts accordingly.

It is interesting to note that in the very successful television shows of the *Marcus Welby* type (the successful and beloved physician, close to Jung's archetype of the Great Healer), the patient almost invariably not only recovers from his physical impairment, but also shows a fundamental and positive change of life-style and attitude. This clearly suggests to the audience that the physical condition will not recur. The patients of *Trapper John, M.D.* generally emerge from the hospital far different people from what they were when they went into it. The television doctor is both a sickness specialist and a health specialist. He (almost invariably the doctor is male) is also the personal physician we all want. (Readers in middle age and beyond will remember how carefully Lionel Barrymore trained young Dr. Kildare to see his patients as complete human beings and respond to their total life, not just to their illness.)

Our actual experiences in the hospital (and with the medical and medical ancillary professions generally) are often, however, far different from the television models. Trained to be an active and aggressive fighter against disease, strongly influenced by the mechanical model of Western civilization, part of a culture that 300 years ago separated the mind from the body (see chapter 2), working with the basic philosophy that made for so much progress in the century just past—that there is *one* cause for each disease and therefore *one* right medical procedure to use (and that the correct diagnosis of the disease is the most crucial factor)—the physician often—quite logically in terms of these conditions—responds to his patients in a manner more suited to a defective mechanism than a suffering person.

A number of years ago, I went on rounds with one of the outstanding neurologists in the world. A group of us, men and women, some in white clothes, some dressed as civilians, went from bed to bed in the wards while the neurologist examined each patient, read from the chart, and described the medical situation to the group. He did not address any of the patients. One patient was a man in his late seventies. With the group crowding around the bed, the neurologist pulled down the sheets, pulled up the man's hospital gown, exposing his genital area, and, pointing to his groin and abdomen, made some comments. After a few moments, the patient, obviously embarrassed, started to pull his gown down. Without pausing in his talk, the doctor pushed his hand away and the gown back up.

This expert and experienced neurologist—seeing the patient as a machine—clearly had no idea that he was lowering the patient's ability to fight his illness and to bring his own self-healing abilities to the aid of the medical treatment. A motor works just as well whether you pat it or spit on it. A person does not, but the doctor was clearly not aware of this.

One patient stated very well her feelings about the mechanical attitude of her physician. An angiogram had been prescribed. In this procedure a long, thin tube is inserted into an artery in the arm and carefully pushed up the artery until the end of it is inside the heart and the heart and the coronary arteries can be dyed and photographed. When this procedure was described to the patient, she felt—even as you and I would—some anxiety and expressed a desire to meet and talk with the specialist who would perform the actual work. Her cardiologist said, "You don't have to know the person who does this. We are all good technicians here." The patient answered, "But I am not an automobile."

One noted psychologist wrote:

I was once in a patient's room, interviewing him informally about his background and current preoccupations, and on several occasions nurses entered the room to perform various "nursing functions." ... This man was seriously ill and had much on his mind, but the nurses came in talking cheerfully and did not cease the

cheerful discourse until they had left. I had little doubt
that the nurses knew no more about this man after they
left than they had when they entered. I verified this
guess when I later asked the nurse to tell me about Mr.
Jones. One nurse replied, "Oh he's a nice fellow." The
other told me, "He's O.K., though sometimes he's a bit
difficult." I asked both of them if they had any idea of
what Mr. Jones had on his mind, and each said that as
far as she knew, he was cheerful most of the time.

George Engel has pointed out that:

Medicine's crisis stems from the logical inference that
since "disease" is defined in terms of somatic param-
eters, physicians need not be concerned with psychosocial issues which lie outside medicine's responsibility
and authority.

A book on dying in our culture reports:

A seventy-eight-year-old man was admitted to a mid-
western teaching hospital for treatment of a bowel ob-
struction. He believed that he was dying, but no one
would listen. When his elderly roommate, suffering
from cancer of the colon, was unsuccessfully resuscitat-
ed while naked and lying in a pool of excretions, the
patient frantically implored the doctor: "Please don't
ever do that to me. Promise that you won't ever do
that to me."

Three days later the patient developed congestive
heart failure and was intubated, placed on a ventilator
and monitored with electrodes on his chest and arms,
all against his will. During the first night of ventilator
care, the patient was found dead in bed. He had awak-
ened, reached over, and switched off the ventilator. On
the bedside table, the doctor found a scribbled note:
"Death is not the enemy, doctor, inhumanity is."

Unfortunately, the attitude that "death is the enemy" is inherent in one of the two major philosophies of curing that exist in modern medicine. A disease-oriented philosophy states that the physician should aggressively "treat the disease in the body in the bed." This approach *has* produced very beneficial results, and no one would suggest that it be discontinued as a mistake. However, it badly needs tempering with a philosophy oriented to the needs and capabilities of each individual person, where each is seen as different, with different needs, capabilities, and feelings.

It would be only too easy to continue with examples of lack of human understanding on the part of physicians and other hospital staff. Every person with experience as a patient or practitioner in the healing field knows a goodly number of them. To continue, however, would obscure two facts.

First, that there is a sizable percentage of physicians and ancillary medical personnel who have always *cared* for their patients and responded to them as suffering individuals. These men and women have been able to stand against their medical training and the strong cultural pressures that equate patients with broken machines.

Second, we are in a period of very rapid change. The view is fast developing that *both* orientations are needed and that medicine must do more than "treat the disease in the body in the bed." Typical of what is going on is the following paragraph from one of the major new textbooks for physicians:

> . . . it makes no sense to talk about functional conditions and organic conditions as being two totally separate entities. We know better. Mind and body are intertwined in a manner which we do not understand, but which nonetheless is indisputable. We must, therefore, view illness not only as a consequence of specific etiologic agents, but also as a consequence of the patient's natural defenses failing to ward off disease. These defenses in-

clude the strength of the patient's spirit, as well as one's antibody levels and the friskiness of one's leukocytes. In order to treat disease, one must therefore attempt to restore and maximize psychic host-resistance and recruit the patient's energy and spirit into the treatment process. To be able to use such resources effectively, the physician must have some understanding of the patient as a person, as well as the circumstances of his or her life situation, before, during, and after treatment.

The University of Pennsylvania Medical Center now has a relaxation specialist working full time in the radiology department. The first army nutritionist, a lieutenant colonel, is now working in Walter Reed Army Medical Center. One of the most rapidly developing fields in modern medicine is that of Family Practice, in which the physician is trained to deal with the whole patient and to treat him over an entire lifetime.

George Engel and his research team, working with sick individuals, have changed the primary questions asked by physicians. Instead of focusing on "What is the cause of this illness?" they have been asking, "Why does *this* patient have *this* disease *now*?" In thus focusing on the *context* of illness, they and others like them are making large strides in a new direction.

A physician writing in what is possibly the most prestigious medical journal printed today—*Lancet*—discusses how important it is for patients to be knowledgeable about their conditions, to make their own decisions, and to keep their treatment and their destiny under their own control. The author goes on to say:

All honour to those who have the courage of their convictions. I include in their number the patients who have gone out of hospital against my advice. I have seen them pioneer the modern treatment of . . . many . . . diseases. I would pay special tribute to the casualties; but the funny thing is that I can't remember any.

In West Germany, one cannot obtain government funds for a cancer clinic or service unless psychological services are also offered. Two years ago, I was between trains in a medium-size Yugoslavian city. While strolling around, I came upon a large hospital of a size that indicated it to be the major one in the area. I thought I would try to look at their cancer service, to see how it differed from those in America, and made my way to the office of the Director of Oncology to ask for permission to wander around. His secretary told me, "I am afraid you will have to wait for an hour. He is tied up right now, leading a group psychotherapy session with our patients."

An extremely knowledgeable specialist in the problems of modern medicine, John H. Knowles, wrote:

A program to improve the self-care of patients with diabetes (tertiary prevention) at the University of Southern California resulted in a 50 percent reduction in emergency-ward visits, a decrease in the number of patients with diabetic coma from 300 to 100 over a two-year period, and the avoidance of 2,300 visits for medication. . . . Savings were estimated at $1.7 million.

Other programs now under way have had much the same type of effect. Returning autonomy to the patient has dramatic positive effects on the patient, the financial system, and the medical load, and is proving to be eminently practical in every respect.

One well-known and accepted text on the sociology of medicine (*Urban Health in America*) lists six objectives as an agenda for health. The third is "a social environment that favors the development of human potential." The sixth— and last—"effective personal health care, provided by competent and interested persons." This order of priorities, which would have been unheard of a few years ago, demonstrates the extent and depth of the new understanding that is developing. (The first objective is "a physical environment that will protect and support human life." The second is "freedom from serious infectious diseases.")

A booklet put out by the World Health Organization in Geneva, "Potential and Development of Traditional Medicine," recommends that mainline medicine examine, learn from, and integrate the medical methods developed in societies other than our own. It stresses the value of these "traditional medicine forms" when used in conjunction with modern Western medical techniques.

There is a new *readiness* to learn in the air. Physicians as well as nonphysicians are becoming more open to new ideas and concepts in health and disease. Typical of the new kinds of things that are happening in the medical field is a report by Robert Swearingen, M.D., who is an orthopedist in private practice in Summit County, Colorado (wonderful skiing country and therefore a place where an orthopedist is going to get a lot of practice setting broken bones), and who is responsible for the Colorado Health Institute in Denver, which deals with preventive medicine and wellness. ("Wellness" meaning a positive movement toward greater health, not just a curing of disease.) Among other additions to the usual mainline medical program, the Institute has a nutritionist and a Department of Life-Style Profiling where all aspects of the client's life are explored for satisfactions, stresses, and deficiencies. Swearingen has described the experience in which he first began really to expand his view of medicine, to "break the shell" of the narrower viewpoint that he had been taught in medical school:

A manifestation of this indignancy from the universe happened one day when I went up to the emergency room to take care of a dislocated shoulder. I did eighty of those, associated with skiing, every winter. I walked in and there was this young man lying on the operating table. I looked at his shoulder and there was an anterior dislocation. I walked back and put my hand on the gentleman's elbow and started pulling some traction down, as it usually decreases the pain. I called out "Nurse!" No one came. Usually there's someone around, nurse, X-ray technician, or someone. So I called again "Nurse!" Still no one came. At that time Aspen was a very small hospital and I could lean over and look down the hall. There was a lot of activity and it turned out later that they had a cardiac arrest. It became obvious that I wasn't going to get a nurse. I needed one to bring me the medication that I was going to put in the vein to relax this person. What you do is move the shoulder and elbow in a certain way and the arm goes back in place, and though the patient may fuss a little bit, he usually doesn't remember much. But I wasn't going to get the medication, which I believed to be a prerequisite to fixing the shoulder. The situation was that of sitting there with some pressure being pulled down on the elbow and the realization that I, as a healing entity, felt totally dependent on technological tools; that I did not feel much strength within myself as an individual to deal with a medical situation without the technological tools. I reached out my other hand and I just set it down on this young man's shoulder as a comforting gesture, and I was amazed that the muscles relaxed. I felt the elbow slide down a little bit. I looked down at him and he was looking up at me with this unbelievable look of trust that only happens in a situation like this. So I explained to him that the medication wasn't coming but that I would stop doing what I was doing if he had any pain. I kept massaging the muscles and asking him to relax and promised him I wouldn't do anything that hurt. He did relax, the elbow came down, the shoulder externally rotated and went right back in place. He had no pain and he had no pain medication.

I was overwhelmed. That was a large egg that had just been broken. There was a belief system that really shook the basic foundations that I had as a physician. I decided it was probably a fluke. Listen, I was comfortable in that eggshell. It was nice, I knew it, it had served me well. It was easier to tell myself it was a fluke. Why take a chance out there where it's scary? But it worked the next time, and the next time, and then they accused me of doing some hocus-pocus! So I taught a resident how to do it and he did it. I had only one person it didn't work on. Yes—another doctor. My belief system wasn't quite as strong as his belief system that it wouldn't work—so it didn't.

The Wellness Clinic at Walter Reed Army Medical Center exemplifies the best aspects of what a health clinic of the future might be like. Headed by Lieutenant Colonel Ray Stephens, it has three major approaches:

1. To teach people to stay well. Individuals who are not sick and wish to increase their level of wellness are helped to evaluate their lives and to determine in what areas they are not nourishing themselves. They are then helped to design programs in terms of their individual needs. These programs may include nutrition, meditation, psychotherapy, exercise, work changes, spiritual development, creativity expansion, and so forth. The emphasis is on helping each participant in the program achieve a unique balance of body, mind, and spirit.

2. To help chronically ill individuals to adapt the disease to their life rather than their life to the disease, and to help them move toward wellness. This in-

cludes such areas as teaching them to recognize in what a small part of their life and body pain actually exists and the differences between pain, pain behavior (what you do in response to pain), and suffering. (In the viewpoint of the Wellness Clinic, "suffering" here refers to resistance to pain and disease that renders people dysfunctional.)

3. To help individuals who are not responding to medical treatment to bring more of their own resources and self-healing abilities to the aid of the medical program. A typical example of this work is shown in the following case history from their files.

R.J. sustained a compound fracture of his left arm in a motorcycle accident. The bone was rather severely shattered. Extensive surgery was done to place all the available fragments together again. After all the pieces were fitted together again, there was nearly half an inch distance between the two ends of the bone. The surgeons placed a steel rod in the arm to give it stability and told R.J. that it was possible, but not probable, that the bone could grow back together.

Three months passed with no bone growth. R.J. came to the Wellness Center at Walter Reed and asked for help. Chaplain S. did not promise anything, but worked out a meditation regime for R.J. and included images that made significant use of R.J.'s rather dynamic faith.

In one month, the half inch of missing bone had grown back, and the bone appeared, on X-ray, to have almost completely mended. However, considerable stiffness had developed in the shoulder and elbow. The focus of meditation was changed to increase the range of motion and to loosen the tight joints.

The primary physician remained skeptical of the influence of meditation on the healing, and Chaplain S. did not claim the meditation practice caused the healing.

However, it was the only difference in the treatment regimen from the time of the break to the present.

When the chaplain and the physician discussed this
case, the physician remained skeptical, but said, "We
have another man with the same problem, maybe you
can help him, too."

As part of the revolution now going on, even house
calls, that strange custom from a long-vanished past, are
making a comeback. In many cities, if you don't think it is a
good idea to take your child who has a temperature of 103°
out on a freezing cold day, you can arrange to have a physician visit you. Special service groups like Medcalls in New
York City or House Calls, Inc., in Portland, Oregon, are now
available. You give your name, age, and symptoms to a
counselor when you call a group. Shortly after, a physician
calls you back and takes the medical details and makes ar-
rangements to visit. The next day you will probably receive
a follow-up phone call to make sure everything went
smoothly, and to see if you have further problems. A medical report will be sent to your regular physician or health
clinic. (You can check with your local medical society to
see if there is a similar service in your own area.)

What is changing today at so rapid a rate is the general
climate of acceptance toward the holistic viewpoint. The
viewpoint itself is nothing new. Many physicians and other
healing professionals have always used it. A dentist like Paul
Krooks of New York City has for many years now observed
the four major tenets of holistic medicine. He views his patients as existing in many interacting domains and refers
them, as advisable, to nutritionists, psychotherapists, and
physicians; he is aware of, and cooperates with, the patient's self-healing and self-repair systems and actively inter-
venes when advisable; he makes sure his patients are
knowledgeable about their dental condition and that they
play an active and decisive role in the decision-making pro-

cess; and he treats each patient as a unique individual. These four concepts are the basic principles of holistic medicine, and many physicians, dentists, and psychotherapists have been following them for a very long time.

In the past, they were a small minority. Today they are in a larger minority, and every indication points to the fact that in the near future a larger percentage of them will be practicing from this orientation. Or—perhaps in most cases—they will be practicing as disease specialists working closely with a health specialist and thus bringing a more complete approach to the medical care of the patient.

THE MECHANIC AND THE GARDENER: TWO APPROACHES TO DISEASE AND HEALTH

As part of the vast ferment going on in Western medicine today, there is a strong and growing recognition of the need to reexamine traditional concepts and definitions. All over America "holistic" and "humanistic" physicians, clinics, and theories are springing up. A great many lay persons are rejecting mainline medicine, in part or in whole, and are trying to solve illness and health problems with a wide variety of techniques ranging all the way from intelligent and carefully thought-out approaches to those based on outright kookiness. These techniques include nutrition, homeopathy, the devouring of vast amounts of vitamins, chanting, meditation, foot massage, the wearing of copper bracelets while sitting under pyramid-shaped structures, psychic healing, acupuncture, yoga, and many others. So angry and rejecting have some of these people become that they have forgotten Eisenbud's First Theorem: "Just because an idea has been rejected by modern science does not mean that ipso facto it is valid."

The ancient Greek historian Herodotus described an experiment that had been done in a Persian city he visited. For one year, the authorities kept track of all patients treated by physicians and how they responded to the accepted medical techniques. Then they exiled the physicians for the following year and built a shaded portico in the center of town. All those who were sick would come there every day or have their relatives carry them there. Passersby were encouraged to talk with a sick person about his symptoms and to discuss their own ideas on the subject. The experiences of others they had known with the same symptoms would be recounted, along with the remedies that had been undertaken. The patients were free to follow any advice they wished. At the end of the year the city authorities compared the results of the two test periods (this was probably the first "controlled" medical experiment in recorded history) and decided to make the exile of the physicians permanent!

In their anger and disillusionment with modern medicine, many people would likely feel that perhaps the ancient Persians had a worthwhile idea. However, anyone who looks at the comparative mortality rates in the Persian empire (or any society before our present one) and the modern era would quickly see the fallacy of this concept.

The revolution in Western medicine has gone much farther than is generally realized. Physicians and nurses are studying and practicing psychic healing. Prestigious medical journals are printing articles on how to laugh your way to health, and Walter Reed Army Medical Center is holding intensive seminars on holistic and humanistic approaches in medicine.

The most conservative bastions of traditional medicine are questioning their own assumptions and experimenting with change.

In order to understand what is going on in medicine today, it is necessary to examine a basic conflict that has been continually fought in this field for at least 2,500 years. This is the problem of what the physician primarily should try to do. Should he actively and forcefully *intervene* when the patient is ill by the use of surgery and strong medicaments to *conquer* the disease? Or should he instead concentrate on finding ways to support the patient's natural healing processes? In effect, should he be primarily a *mechanic* and repair the ill body, or should he be primarily a *gardener* and help the body grow past disease and toward health?

It would be foolish to argue that the physician should be completely one or the other. Both roles are clearly necessary. The most mechanically oriented surgeon is aware that the best sutures in the world can only bring the sides of the wound together in such a way that healing can take place and the patient's self-recuperative abilities can seal it. The most fervid "natural healing" devotee would agree that if an artery is cut and spouting blood, a surgical intervention is needed immediately.

Medicine is not and never has been a matter of one extreme or another. The question of emphasis, however, is extremely important and the front lines of the battle have surged back and forth since at least the time of Hippocrates. Indeed, his is the first clear statement espousing one side or the other that we possess. He saw disease as being made up of two elements—suffering (*Pathos*) and restitutive healing attempts of the body (*Ponos*)—and believed the physician should primarily search for, try to understand, and aid the *Ponos*. Reporting this, the twelfth-century physician Maimonides wrote:

> Galen has already explained to us that the ancient Greeks, when in doubt as to what to do in a certain disease, did nothing but left the patient to Nature, which they considered sufficient to cure all illnesses. . . . And it is true that the physician should help Nature, support it and do nothing else but follow it.

In Roman times, the conflict between those who believed in the healing powers of the body and in cooperating with them (the Hippocratics), and those who believed that this passive approach was useless, a mere "meditation on death," and that active intervention was necessary (the followers of Asclepiades of Bithynia), continued with violent argument and vituperation on both sides.

The idea that much of what is perceived as "illness" is

due to the body's actions of a restorative and self-healing nature was not lost after the classical period, but also was typical of the medieval approach. Thus according to the Theory of Humors (the accepted medical theory of the period) it was believed that illness was due to an excess of one of the four kinds of fluid in the body and that, when this condition occurred, certain self-healing dispositions of the body automatically went into action. For example, these dispositions raised the body temperature so as to "cook" the excess of raw fluid and then separate the cooked from the uncooked parts. The physician *cooperated* with these self restorative dispositions. He gave warming drinks and warmed the patient externally to help with the cooking. He then helped the body to dispose of the cooked excess by giving purges and emetics and by bleeding. Thus, from his viewpoint, every disease was a process which the physician could help regulate by cooperating with the self-healing abilities of the patient.

According to the sixteenth-century physician Paracelsus, "Man is his own doctor and finds healing herbs in his own garden. The physician is in ourselves, and in our own nature are all the things we need."

In Paracelsus' day, medicine was divided between the "Galenic" physicians, who favored herbal preparations intended to cooperate with the body's healing efforts, and the "Spagyric" physicians, who favored the use of chemical preparations intended to intervene actively in the process of the disease. The comments they made about each other were very similar to the comments made by the opponents of "holistic" and "mainline" medicine today.

Once the Church permitted dissection of human beings for medical purposes in the seventeenth century, it reinforced the idea, already developing in the philosophy of the period, that body and mind were separate and should be considered separately. The background for the Cartesian dualism of our time was greatly strengthened. The physical body could be dissected and investigated by anatomists; the soul and mind remained the province of theology and philosophy. Since the body and the mind had been separated by the Church, and since the science of the time was mechanical, the belief took hold that the body itself was a machine, disease a consequence of the breakdown of this machine, and the physician's task was mechanical repair of the parts.

Descartes formally stated this view, and it achieved wide popularity.

> Descartes's ... description effectively turned the human body into a clockworks and placed a new distance, not only between mind and body, but also between the patient's complaint and the physician's eye. Within this mechanized framework, pain turned into a red light and sickness into mechanical trouble. A taxonomy of diseases became possible. ... Instead of suffering man, sickness was placed in the center of the medical system. ...

Medicine increasingly adopted the view that the physician's task was actively to intervene in and conquer disease. Gradually the idea that the body had self-healing abilities was lost. Some physicians tried to restore the older viewpoint or to strike a balance, but they were unsuccessful.

Thomas Sydenham, in the seventeenth century, tried in vain to recall his profession to the idea that, in the words of one historian, "nature, rightly understood and left to herself, was perhaps the best healer." Against the rising tide of a mechanistic view of the cosmos and of man, however, even Sydenham was helpless. He set himself the task of challenging Descartes's concept of men as automata and machinery. He wrote clearly and well and had an immense prestige, but to no avail.

Throughout Europe and America in the eighteenth century, medical opinion was primarily on the side of active intervention against disease. The physician saw himself as the

enemy of the disease process and his task to take arms
against it. However, his knowledge and tools were as scant
and ineffective as ever, and neither he nor those who es-
poused the "natural" healing methods were able to do
much good. Neither school knew very much and, what was
worse, most of what they were sure they knew was wrong.
The "naturopaths" probably obeyed to a much greater degree Hippocrates' "First Law" (*Primum non nocere*: Above
all, do no harm) because they acted less aggressively and
their remedies were weaker. It may be that this is the reason
that in the early 1800s public opinion began to favor their
approach.

On one side was the Popular Health Movement (PHM)
and on the other the orthodox physicians. The PHM used
mostly plant and herb remedies and attacked the mainline
physicians for their "barbaric" treatments, their fees, and
their "arrogance." They sought to "return medicine to the
people," to "make every man his own doctor," partly
through Samuel Thompson's "Friendly Botanical Societies."
Opposing them were many leading physicians such as the
French F.J.U. Broussais, who believed only active measures
could cure disease since the body had no natural healing
power. In the event, the PHM and its allies were so successful that in the United States, state after state repealed its laws
licensing physicians, and by 1849 only New Jersey and the
District of Columbia had such laws still on the books. It
would seem that the "intervene and conquer" viewpoint in
medicine was in full rout.

Many physicians of the period also believed that there
should be a wider approach to the healing arts than mainline medicine could provide. Benjamin Rush, who was Surgeon General of the United States Army (and a signer of the
Declaration of Independence), wrote:

> The Constitution of this Republic should make special
> provision for Medical Freedom as well as Religious Free-
> dom. . . . To restrict the art of healing to one class of

men and deny equal privileges to others will constitute
the Bastille of medical science. All such laws are un-
American and despotic.

However, during the course of the next century the picture was completely reversed. With two major advances in
medicine, the physicians' ability to intervene successfully
against and cure disease became greater than at any other
time in history. Germ theory and the consequent introduction of antiseptic surgery on the one hand, and medicine's
alliance with the new science of chemistry on the other, led
to a dramatic new control of many heretofore deadly diseases. Communicable and infectious diseases such as tuberculosis, smallpox, and typhus were largely brought under
control. The Sanitary Revolution of the late 1800s in which
the water supply was improved, housing laws were passed,
linen underclothing became more popular (it was much
easier to wash than the older woolen underclothes and so
was likely to be changed more often), and a public *attitude*
toward cleanliness developed, played a large part, but so
did vaccination and a host of other medical techniques.
Work such as that of Lister changed hospitals from places
where if what caused you to go there did not kill you, the
infections you contracted there almost certainly would, to
places where the benefits of being there vastly outweighed
the risks. The Flexner Report of 1910 completely reorganized American hospitals and made them into incompara-
bly better treatment centers than the world had ever
seen before.

The conflict between the Galenic and the Spagyric physicians that had begun in the sixteenth century continued
into the twentieth. At that time, the great pharmaceutical
houses realized that for them there was an immense advantage in chemical medications. Unlike natural medicaments,
they could be patented. The development of chemistry permitted the synthesis of many natural products in the labora-

tory. Not only could they be better standardized if made in this way, but, being patentable, they could be the source of large amounts of money. A massive promotional effort was made by the new pharmaceutical houses to convince the general population that chemical products were superior to natural products. This effort was largely successful. In the nation's medicine cabinets, herbs gave way to their synthetic correlates.

Since 1800, mainline medicine has been based largely on an ancient idea known as the Doctrine of Contraries. The idea is so simple and obvious that it has come to be thought of as the most basic common sense. Anyone questioning it is thought to be simpleminded or fanatical.

The medical writer Brian Inglis described the doctrine simply: ". . . that where the body's working deviated from the normal, a counteracting procedure should be applied. Thus, a man suffering from constipation would be given a laxative; if he was feverish, ways would be found to cool him, and so on."

When germs were discovered to be implicated in many diseases, the idea seemed validated. If the germs were eliminated, the disease could be cured. If the patient had a deviation from the normal—the presence of specific bacteria—the physician had only to attack and destroy them and the disease would be cured.

This concept has certainly produced tremendous progress in many areas and ended the threat of many diseases. However, it blocked understanding of two major factors: first, the patient's own self-healing ability, and the fact that many symptoms (deviations from the normal) are the result of the restitutive attempts of the body—the Hippocratic *Ponos*. Second, that many patients with the bacteria present in their systems did not develop the disease; that the "single cause" concept of disease, although sometimes fruitful, was always false.

One reason that we retain the one-factor theory of disease (each disease is due to one factor, one germ, one virus, and so on) is that it simplifies matters and makes problems easier to deal with. In 1979 there was an epidemic among the slum children of Naples, Italy, who began dying of a fulminating viral infection. Everyone agreed that only those children living in the slums were dying. The experts in Naples immediately got in touch with the Communicable Disease Center in Atlanta, Georgia, and set up an attempt to discover a vaccine. Think how this orientation simplifies matters. You ignore the big question of why the virus does a right about-face every time it comes to the edge of a slum and stays away from the children in suburbs. You do not have to worry about problems such as decent food and housing, breathable air, etc. Social problems are tough ones. The idea that one virus equals one disease makes it possible to ignore them.

(This resembles our insistent clinging to the mechanistic view of the universe. One reason we hang on to it—in the face of a storm of contrary evidence—is that it is the simplest and least mind-straining view of how things work that we humans have ever developed. It may not be valid, at least for large stretches of experience, but it *is* simple.)

The one-factor theory is gradually dying in medicine. More and more physicians are coming to the viewpoint that disease and health are problems not just of cells but of the total human organism: that *people* contract disease and that people must be dealt with in resolving medical and health problems. Typical of this new understanding is the formation of such organizations as Physicians for Social Responsibility (PO Box 411, New York, NY 10024) sponsored by physicians of impeccable prestige and position such as Helen Caldicott, Jerome Frank, Herbert Abrams, Sidney Alexander, and a host of others.

The falsity of the "single cause" premise has been shown in dramatic highlight by its inapplicability to the degenerative diseases. In spite of vast and very expensive research projects, no single cause for these diseases has ever been found or is likely to be. Farmers who have never smoked and who live in the clean air of the country do develop lung cancer; athletes who have a very low cholesterol level do have heart attacks; multiple sclerosis strikes apparently at random.

Holistic medicine rejects the single-cause theory of disease. It is based on the belief that the patient must be seen as existing on many, equally important levels, and that steps should be taken against the disease and toward the development of health on as many of these as possible. Further, for each patient, an individual and unique combination of going "contrary" to the disease, and of stimulating the patient's resistance to it and his growth toward health, must be designed.

It is true that many practitioners of the adjunctive modalities that are today loosely grouped under the term "holistic medicine" do not understand these basic principles and believe that working on the particular level they are interested in is all that is important. Those who cling to just one of these modalities to the exclusion of all others are, in fact, using the theories of mainline medicine that they constantly criticize, but with a technique that mainline medicine does not recognize as effective.

In mainline medicine itself, there has been little exploration or criticism of the basic philosophical ideas on which the craft is based. Nor is there any evidence of interest in such exploration. The New York Academy of Medicine, for example, has one of the great medical libraries of the world. It subscribes to hundreds of well-known and obscure medical journals. *The Journal of Medical Philosophy* is not one of them. As Inglis puts it:

> Although occasionally an elder statesman in the profession has been permitted to sound a warning or a querulous note, articles questioning the whole basis of

orthodox medicine have been almost as unusual in medical journals as objections to the doctrine of Papal infallibility in *L'Osservatore Romano*.

It is no new thing for medicine to be conservative and resistant to new ideas. The term *dogmatic* comes from the name of a society formed by the sons and son-in-law of Hippocrates. They were attempting to protect patients against the damaging effects of new and untried theories and medications. Their view was that the writings of Hippocrates formed the final word possible in medicine and that neither new ideas nor new procedures were acceptable.

It is important to understand that resistance to new ideas in medicine has not only the usual conservative dynamics of every art and science behind it, but also a desire to protect the patient. Usually, as we all know, this conservatism goes much too far. It is unfortunate that in one area at least it has not gone far enough. This is in the area of the relationship between the physician and the drug company. Generally holding a deep belief in modern science and medical progress, physicians tend to trust the products put out by the pharmaceutical houses on the say-so of their advertisements. (That anyone should, in this age, trust a large company to be interested in anything but making money boggles the imagination!) And with the tremendous flood of medical information constantly being published in literally hundreds of professional journals, many physicians find themselves relying on the summaries and other reports put out by the drug companies about their own products. Once a product has been marketed, the drug companies tend to resist information about negative side effects, the fact it does not accomplish its purpose, and so on, until the last moment when they are faced with lawsuits or the Federal Drug Administration is about to move. A typical case of this sort was the Dalcron Shield, an intrauterine contraceptive device that has made a large number of women sterile. The drug company involved did very little testing, did not heed warnings from its own consultants, and even after it stopped manufacturing the IUD a few years ago (and was being faced with more than forty lawsuits) did not withdraw the million-plus devices still on the market.

It is unfortunate that the official medical organizations do not hold a tighter rein on the drug companies. It has been suggested by many people that one reason for this is that the largest part of the over $240 million a year that the drug companies spend on advertising is spent for space in medical journals, which would have a very hard time continuing to publish without this income. Probably of more importance, however, is the fact that physicians are like the rest of us in this culture. They believe in progress so strongly that they trust the claims of advertisers.

The idea that a remedy for each disease existed in natural form if it could only be found has changed in this century, with a deep faith in science replacing the older faith in nature. The beginning of this change was marked by the discovery by the chemist Ehrlich in 1909 of Salvarsan, a manufactured drug to treat syphilis. (It was called "606" at the time, as it was the six hundred and sixth compound in the series Ehrlich developed.) Instead of hoping we might discover a specific plant or herb to cure each disease, we now waited, with firm conviction that it would happen, for the drug companies to develop an *artificial* substance that would be specific for each disease.

Indeed, many such specifics were developed, including remedies for such conditions as amoebic dysentery, malaria, sleeping sickness, and blood poisoning. As the surgeon-philosopher Kenneth Walker wrote: "... The partnership between the chemists and the doctors is proving to be one of the most profitable partnerships in the whole history of medicine."

One has only to read the accounts of the ancient chroniclers of the epidemics that ravaged their world to realize how much the sanitary revolution of the late nineteenth century, and the medical advances of the nineteenth and twentieth centuries, have contributed to our welfare. When we read about the hopelessness that people felt as Athens, Rome, Byzantium, and the rest of the classical and medieval worlds were ravaged again and again, of how entire sections of the world were depopulated, of how the course of history was changed by diseases with mysterious and terrible effects, we can begin to sense how far we have come.

The Byzantine historian Procopius described the great plague of the era of Justinian which started in A.D. 521.

> During these times there was a pestilence, by which the whole human race came near to being annihilated. . . . For it did not come in a part of the world nor upon certain men, nor did it confine itself to any season of the year, so that from such circumstances it might be possible to find subtle explanations of a cause, but it embraced the entire world, and blighted the lives of all men, though differing from one another in a most marked degree, respecting neither sex nor age . . . it left neither island nor cave nor mountain ridge which had human inhabitants. . . . Death came in some cases immediately, in others after many days. . . . Indeed the whole matter may be stated thus, that no device was discovered by man to save himself, so that either by taking precautions he should not suffer, or that when the malady had assailed him he should get the better of it; but suffering came without warning. . . .

So dramatic were the results of the new techniques for treating disease that the experiences which told the practicing physician that each patient was different in his susceptibility and his response to bacterial or other infection, or to any other disease process, were overlooked in medical training. Generation after generation of physicians graduated from medical school trained to look only at the specific disease, and not to be concerned with the ill patient. Individual differences among patients were largely forgotten, as were the patient's own self-healing abilities. Spurred on by the tremendous public prestige the medical profession had gained by its new skills, and by the belief that physicians had, or were developing in the laboratories, the skills finally to conquer disease altogether, medical schools ignored both the warnings of many outstanding experienced physicians about, and the actual hard evidence of, the limitations to their single-minded approach.

There were both warnings and contrary evidence in plentiful supply. Claude Bernard, one of the great medical researchers of the nineteenth century, wrote: "Illnesses hover constantly about us, their seeds blown by the wind, but they do not set in the terrain unless the terrain is ready to receive them."

And Pasteur's last words were widely reported to be: "Bernard is right. The germ is nothing; the terrain all."

Around 1900 a number of scientists drank glasses of cultures isolated from fatal cases of cholera. Tremendous numbers of cholera vibrios could be found in their stools: none developed true cholera. More recently volunteers ingested dysentery bacilli under ideal conditions for infection (enteric capsules full of feces taken directly from people with bacillary dysentery were used) and very few developed the disease. The *context* of disease was missed by the famous experiments of Pasteur and Koch, who found the ideal animals for infection, the ideal vectors for infecting them, but ignored the "terrain."

In the Lübeck Catastrophe of 1926, 249 babies were accidentally injected with tremendous doses of tuberculosis bacilli. Thirty-five percent died from acute TB, but 65 percent survived and were found to be free of disease twelve years later.

Experiments with cancer have produced the same results. Injecting cancer-free volunteers with live cancer cells—as has been done in some studies recently—does not produce cancer. It produces a local irritation at the point of injection that very soon clears up by itself. If you wish to use animals for experimentation, you either have to use carefully bred animals that genetically have a very weak cancer defense mechanism, or else must pretreat your animals with radiation or something of the sort to weaken the animals' defense.

The epidemiologist Richard Doll has pointed out that even powerful carcinogenic agents do not necessarily cause cancer. There were 2,500 residents of Hiroshima and Nagasaki who were less than 1,100 meters from ground zero and survived. Less than 2 percent developed leukemia—a figure high enough to show the leukogenic effects of radiation, but low enough to show the importance of other factors.

The Wall Street Journal (August 25, 1980) reported that over a six-year period a 1 percent rise in unemployment causes 37,000 deaths. The incidence of virtually all major diseases and all major causes of death are increased, including infant mortality, suicide, heart disorders, stroke, liver conditions, and automobile accidents. We see, in this type of statistic, the clear indication that one cannot separate the "terrain" and the specific cause of death.

In the cases of infants who received insufficient mothering, loving, and touching, the death rates were very high. Their illness was called "marasmus" by Margaret Ribble and "anaclitic depression" by René Spitz, but they did not die of this. Their illness was a generalized weakness, an inability to develop, and a susceptibility to a wide variety of specific diseases which killed them. Their bodies' defenses had collapsed and they were vulnerable to whatever bacteria, virus, or developmental fault was present. The same type of reaction was shown in adults by the German sociologist Arthur Jores. He examined the records of a large number of ex-Nazis who had spent their working lives in the German administrative system and were fired under the "denazification" program, and told that they could never be employed in it again. Jores studied particularly those in the thirty-five-to forty-year-old range. Over the next five years their deaths from all causes (including cancer, heart attacks, strokes, accidents) peaked to the death rates usually found in the same employment group between the ages of sixty-five to seventy. (Retirement age in that work was at sixty-five.) After five years, their death rates went back down to those usual for their ages. The assumption was that if they survived that long, they were very likely to have found other jobs and ways of meaningfully living and expressing themselves.

Widowers have a death rate three to five times higher than age-equated married men for all causes of deaths.

A description of a study by psychologists Christeson and Hickle states that:

> In an industrial study in the United States they have shown that managers in a company, who by virtue of their family background and educational experience were least well prepared for the demands and expectations of industrial life, were at greater risk of disease than age-matched managers who were better prepared. They found that this increased risk included all diseases, major as well as minor, physical as well as mental, long-term as well as short-term.

René Dubos has pointed out that "the microbial diseases most common . . . today arise from the activities of microorganisms that are ubiquitous in the environment, present in the body without causing harm under ordinary circumstances. . . ."

We have begun to comprehend how the resistance of the individual to pathogens of all kinds is affected by factors at all levels including the social. This can be experimentally demonstrated, even with animal studies.

> Alteration of the social environment by varying the size of the group in which animals interact, while keeping all

aspects of the physical environment and diet constant, has been reported to lead to the following: a rise in maternal and infant mortality rates; an increase in the incidence of arteriosclerosis; a marked reduction in the resistance to a wide variety of noxious stimuli including drugs, microorganisms and X-rays; an increased susceptibility to various types of neoplasia; alloxan-produced diabetes and convulsions.

In Norman Cousins's words: ". . . the will to live is not a theoretical abstraction, but a physiologic reality with therapeutic characteristics."

The interrelationship between the faith and attitude of the patient and the effects of physical intervention is one of the oldest, most consistently overlooked, and constantly rediscovered pieces of medical knowledge. In the time of Ramses II of Egypt, a medical writer said: "Incantations are excellent for remedies, and remedies are excellent for incantations."

Hippocrates wrote that "it is not enough for us [the physicians] to do what we can do. The patient and his environment and external conditions have to contribute to achieve the cure."

Kenneth Walker could write in the 1950s, "A medicine's value depends almost as much on the patient's faith in it as on what it contains. . . ." And yet the implications of this common knowledge—common to every experienced physician—could be almost completely ignored by medical research in the following years.

Many individual physicians, often widely known and respected ones, saw the dangerous and self-limiting path medicine was on.

In 1927, Francis Peabody wrote in a classic paper:

The most common criticism made at present by older practitioners is that young graduates have been taught a great deal about the mechanism of disease, but very little about the practice of medicine—or, to put it more bluntly—they are too "scientific" and do not know how to take care of patients.

There was much dramatic evidence in the practice of every physician that each patient was different in susceptibility and in response to disease-causing agents. Sir William Osler, one of the greatest and most noted physicians of the early part of the twentieth century, said in a famous and often repeated statement: "It is more important to know what sort of patient has the disease than to know what sort of disease the patient has." But in spite of this evidence, and the warnings to the contrary, the view that "one germ equals one disease," that each disease is caused *only* by a specific bacterium, became more entrenched, and individual differences among patients and the fact that there were restitutive healing processes naturally inherent in the patient were lost sight of.

In the first half of the twentieth century, many medical people realized that the separation of mind and body in diagnosis and treatment had gone too far and was blocking further progress. Out of this realization came the modern field of psychosomatic medicine.

The concept of psychosomatic functioning has been around for a long time. In the year 1402 the physician Maestro Lorenzo Sassoli wrote a letter to a patient of his. In part it read:

> ... let me speak to you regarding the things of which you must be most aware. To get angry and shout at times pleases me, for this will keep up your natural heat; but what displeases me is your being grieved and taking all matters to heart. For it is this, as the whole of medicine teaches, which destroys our body more than any other cause.

In his *Tristram Shandy*, written in the eighteenth century, Laurence Sterne wrote: "Man's body and mind, with the utmost reverence to both I speak it, are exactly like a jerkin and a jerkin's lining; rumple the one and you rumple the other."

The theory of humors, which was the major medical theory of the medieval and Renaissance periods, included a complex and sophisticated psychosomatic viewpoint. Until the seventeenth century there was no real concept of the separation of mind and body. It was only after Descartes that this dualism was accepted. By the end of the nineteenth century, however, the separation had grown to a point that the interaction was not taught and was hardly mentioned in medical training or textbooks. The experience of all observant physicians that mental states affected bodily functioning was ignored.

The developing field of psychiatry in the next fifty years recognized this interaction was of crucial importance in many diseases. Psychiatry, combined with advancing knowledge in physiology and internal medicine, made it clear to many physicians that they could no longer maintain the rigid lines of separation, that medicine and surgery could deal with the specific disease and its symptoms, but that the patient's emotional status would have to be changed if the condition were not to recur.

Under the leadership of psychiatrists like Nolan D. C. Lewis, Gotthard Booth, Flanders Dunbar, and Franz Alexander, and internists like Arnold Hutschnecker, the new field developed rapidly. Although *all* diseases were clearly a function of a complete human being encompassing both mind and body, a rough, working definition was gradually established. A *psychosomatic disease* was—in effect—defined as a disease in which two approaches were known to have an effect on the prognosis: the medical-surgical approach on the one hand, and psychotherapy on the other. Although there were extremists on both sides who advocated the use of just one of these approaches in specific diseases, the general view is that both are necessary for the best treatment.

In this way, psychosomatic medicine became the first medically accepted development in the direction of holistic medicine. The patient was seen as existing on two interacting levels, both of which must be taken into account by the physician. Without psychosomatic medicine, it is extremely doubtful that there would, today, be a holistic medicine movement.

However, psychosomatic practice and theory, although it opened the gate to the present development, stopped short and did not proceed through the gate. Instead of a viewpoint encompassing *all* levels of the person, it added only the emotional to the factors producing disease. In a sense, it added a new continent to medical theory, but not a new cosmos.

One reason that doctors continued to focus primarily on the illness itself was the structure of the modern hospital. With the introduction of accurate methods of measuring various body functions, there was, in the nineteenth century, a shift of interest on the part of the physician. He became better trained to observe (and was therefore more interested in) illness than in persons who were ill. With a detailed classification of illnesses, a sickness became an entity that could be mentally detached from a human being and described as a thing in itself. Hospitals divided themselves into different sections, each corresponding to a group of classifications—"a compartmentalized repair shop." Hospitals became places to treat sickness rather than to treat persons who were ill. (There is, by the way, no evidence that splitting a hospital up into sections corresponding to various aspects of the present classification of disease is helpful to the recovery of patients. The only experiment in this area of which I am aware—that done by Kurt Goldstein in the 1920s—provided evidence in the opposite direction. It is, however, very convenient for the staff and for training personnel to divide a hospital into sections in this way.)

Once we organize a hospital according to diseases or different organ systems, we are subtly (but very strongly) training hospital personnel to think in terms of diseases and organ systems and not in terms of people. As a matter of fact, if you asked a psychologist the best way to train medical personnel to see only the similarity among patients (that is, the illness that they have) and to forget that differences in genetic background, life experience, and attitude exist, the psychologist would almost certainly start by recommending that the patients be grouped separately by their medical classifications and—to the degree possible—kept in separate locations. A ghetto system is as effective a way as we know of building stereotypes so that we cease seeing people as individuals and start seeing them as "Blacks," "Jews," "Catholics," "hearts," "stomachs," or what have you. Our hospital "department" system is one of our most effective ways of retraining medical personnel so that they no longer see and react to their patients as individual human beings, but rather as diseases with people somehow, and rather irrelevantly, attached to them.

The physician Jon Garfield has pointed out in some detail how the Flexner Report of 1910 (which led to a radical revision and restructuring of American hospitals, and which was responsible for their assuming their present form) plus the concept of specific etiology of disease—one cause equals one disease—led to the present training program for physicians, which in turn has resulted in physicians who see the patient as little more than a malfunctioning machine.

It is from this extreme state of affairs that the present ferment in attitudes toward sickness and health has developed. For various reasons, a rising discontent with medical results and a loss in prestige of the physician have been developing in America over the last three decades. (I shall discuss these reasons in some detail in chapter 5.) The public at large and the medical profession itself came to recognize the need to see and react to the patient as an individual organism, functioning as a complete body-mind-spirit environment, rather than as a broken machine to be fixed.

Typical of the best of the new approach is Martin Lipp's *Respectful Treatments: The Human Side of Medical Care.* In this manual for physicians, Lipp teaches expertly and lucidly how to deal with a patient as a full human being and how to avoid responding to him as a disease entity. He shows how the physician can be both disease specialist and health therapist. His patients are *respected* and are involved in their own medical decisions and treatment.

In his presidential address to the American Cancer Society in 1959, Eugene Pendergrass said:

> Anyone who has had extensive experience in the treatment of cancer is aware that there are great differences among patients. . . . I personally have observed cancer patients who have undergone successful treatment and were living and well for years. Then an emotional stress, such as the death of a son in World War II, the infidelity of a daughter-in-law, or the burden of long unemployment, seem to have been precipitating factors in the reactivation of their disease which resulted in death. . . . There is solid evidence that the course of disease in general is affected by emotional distress. . . . Thus, we, as doctors, may begin to emphasize treatment of the patient as a *whole*, as well as the disease from which the patient is suffering. We may learn how to influence general body systems, and through them modify the neoplasm which resides within the body.
>
> As we do go forward . . . searching for new means of influencing growth both within the cell and through systemic influences, it is my sincere hope that we can widen the quest to include the distinct possibility that within one's mind is a power capable of exerting forces

which can either enhance or inhibit the progress of this disease.

Kenneth Walker, in describing the origin of the newly developing views in medicine, wrote:

When we pass in review the various theories of illness put forward in different times in history, we find that they are reflections of philosophy and science prevalent at that time. Because the materialistic and deterministic-minded scientists of the last century interpreted everything in terms of mechanism, it was natural that contemporary medical men should follow their lead and should look upon the sick man as a broken machine. They said that something had gone wrong with his interior mechanism, so that the many wheels of his being no longer moved together harmoniously, and as the new science of pathology advanced, a more exact account of the nature of the mechanism breakdown was offered. It was now said that the patient was ill because his bowel had become obstructed, because a gallstone had lodged in his bile-duct, or because the valves of his heart had been so badly damaged by an attack of rheumatic fever suffered in childhood that they no longer prevented the back-flow of blood into the auricle. Again there was much truth in this broken-machine view of illness, as there had been truth in the previous theory of the four humours, and again the mistake was made of applying the theory too widely. Another error for which this mechanical interpretation of disease was responsible was that it directed the doctor's attention too exclusively to the working of a single organ, so that he often lost sight of the patient as a human whole. The doctor became so engrossed in what he was doing—namely, treating an obstructed bowel, an enlarged liver, or defective cardiac valves—that he entirely forgot the existence of a sen-

tient and very worried man or woman. Now a human
being is much more than a number of organs cleverly
packed into a minimum of space and wrapped around
with a covering of waterproof sheeting. He is a mysterious complex mind, body, and spirit, no one of which
can be disturbed without the rest of him becoming disordered. The broken machinery concept of disease was
therefore that highly dangerous thing, a half-truth mas-
querading as a whole truth, an idea which, followed too
blindly, as the idea of the broken engine was followed
during the nineteenth century, gave rise to a legion of
errors.

The practitioners of the art of medicine have thus been
in conflict over one issue since Roman times at least, and
probably much earlier. Should medicine do as much, and as
actively, as possible, or should it do as little as possible in
order to deal most effectively with the disease? Should it be
King Stork or King Log? Should the physician stress intervention and repair, or should he stress cooperation with the
defenses of the body? Thanks to the tremendous and invaluable development of technology, medicine in the past
hundred years has moved increasingly to the side of active
intervention. We now *can* intervene far more and far more
successfully than ever before. We have an *active* medical
technique of great power for many diseases. But we are beginning to see the limitations of this approach, that without
cooperation with the defenses and repair systems of the
body there are many things we cannot do. Much of the
struggle and ferment in the field of medicine today is due to
this growing realization. We are beginning to comprehend
that *the solution lies not in espousing one approach or the
other, but in finding how best to combine them in an individual manner for each patient.*
What is most important is that we retain a sense of pro-
portion about the problems of illness and of health and not

go to extremes. To dismiss the accomplishments of traditional medicine—as many people in the "holistic" and "humanistic" health field do—is to ignore uncounted hours of dedicated service, of profound study and research, and tremendous medical advances. Lewis Thomas sums up one aspect of this very well when he writes:

> Looking back at the records of infectious disease in Western society over the past two centuries, it is obvious that the incidence of most bacterial diseases began to fall long before the introduction of the sulfonamides and the antibiotics.
>
> The mortality from tuberculosis was halved every twenty years since the mid-nineteenth century, and something like this was happening to pneumonia and streptococcal infections.
>
> This steady improvement in human health has been variously attributed to better sanitation, better nutrition, better housing, less crowding, and a generally better standard of living.
>
> Looking at these events, a number of influential epidemiologists and public-health professionals have suggested that perhaps the impact of chemotherapy on infection was an illusion. We would have gotten where we are today—relatively free from the threat of tuberculosis and other infectious diseases—without scientific medicine, it is said, by allowing society to continue to improve our ways of living together. Fix society, fix the environment, change our life-styles, mend our ways—and human disease will vanish.
>
> If you believe this, you automatically take a different and highly skeptical view not only of the social value of medical science in the past, but also of its prospects for the future. You can get along by abstinence and jogging and maybe a bit of faith healing. It has an undeniable appeal.

My own view of the argument is a totally biased one, but I cannot help this. I have been conditioned by the experience of seeing children with miliary tuberculosis and tuberculous meningitis cured of their illnesses that were by definition 100 percent fatal in my student days, and I saw no reason to doubt my eyes.

I have watched patients with typhoid fever, meningitis, streptococcal septicemia and erysipelas and overwhelming pneumococcal infections get better, sometimes overnight, and I am as certain as I am of my sanity, that these were real events and not illusions.

In short, I haven't any doubt at all as to the effectiveness of today's antibacterial and immunological measures for disease control, although I am worried about the future of antibiotics (as is everyone else in the field of infectious disease) if we do not continue to do research on the appalling problems of antibiotic resistance among our most common pathogens.

In the following chapters, I shall be discussing the present situation in medicine and the potentialities for the future at much greater length. But first it is necessary to look briefly at the tremendous revolution in basic scientific theory that took place after 1900, a revolution that made possible the new concepts in medicine.

THE SCIENTIFIC REVOLUTION OF THE TWENTIETH CENTURY

In the year 1900 a profound revolution in scientific thought took place.* It was a revolution of such dimensions that we are still in its midst and still exploring its implications. Nineteen hundred was the year that Max Planck developed quantum mechanics.

Quantum mechanics is the science by means of which we study and deal with things which are too small ever to see or touch, even with instruments like microscopes. These are the subatomic particles such as electrons or protons. At best we can only see their effects as when one of them passes through a cloud chamber and leaves a visible trail behind it, like a jet plane too far away to see except by its vapor trail. When billions of these particles are forced to interact in a particular way, we can see the result in the mushroom cloud that hangs over our civilization like the sword of Damocles.

What Planck did was to develop useful scientific laws for learning about things which we knew existed, but which were too small to see or touch. The major task of a science has always been to make all kinds of data understandable and to search for laws that fit what we observe.

What Planck found was that the laws in the "quantum realm" are very different from the laws in

*This subject is dealt with at much greater length and detail in L. LeShan, and H. Margenau, *Einstein's Space and Van Gogh's Sky: Physical Reality and Beyond* (New York: Macmillan, 1981)

the realm of everyday experience where we use our senses to perceive and understand the world around us. When things we know exist are too small to see, there is no way to understand them unless we develop a whole new system of explanations for the things that happen. The clear implication of the Planck revolution is that there is *no one way* of explaining everything: different kinds of explanations are needed in different realms of experience.

For the first time a science had been developed to deal with a realm of experience that could not be directly observed and experienced by our human sensory equipment, even with the aid of instruments.

One of the things that the new science demonstrated was that in these other realms, we cannot use a mechanical model. The way of thinking about reality that had proved so fruitful from 1700 to 1900 could not be extended to *all* of reality. According to this earlier way of thinking, a thing can be broken down into its components (as a machine is taken apart into cogs, wheels, levers, and so forth) and its working explained as the sum of the workings of the parts; it can then be reassembled, and it will work as well as before. Things in this sensory realm function in ordinary "yardstick" space and in ordinary "clock" time, and—in short—conform to what we would call "common sense."

The belief that this model of the way things work applied to *all* reality was one of the cornerstones of pre-1900 thinking. It was for this reason that so much progress was made in some areas (those areas of experience accessible to the senses, where the model applied), and so little progress made in some other areas (such areas as the realm of consciousness, where the data are not accessible to the senses and where the model did not apply). The fact that the mechanical model is not applicable to the realm of consciousness has been crucial to the development in our culture of a new approach to the subject of health.

A few years after the discovery of quantum mechanics, Einstein showed that a third system was needed for the realm of experience in which things were very big or were moving—relative to us—very fast. In his theory of relativity, he demonstrated that the explanatory system needed to describe the data from this realm was different from that needed for the realm of the senses and from that needed for the realm of the very small.

For our purposes, in applying these new scientific principles to health and medical care, what we need to understand is that different systems of explanation (rules governing how things work) do not contradict each other; they are compatible. In spite of the fact that one system of rules cannot be applied to everything, each set of rules makes perfect sense if used in the appropriate area. A set of rules that might be ridiculous for driving an automobile might make perfect sense in the realm of the very small, where it is normal for an electron to go from one path (orbit) to another without crossing the space in between. Or to pass through two holes in a screen at the same time without splitting apart. Or in the realm of the very large and fast, the faster an object moves (relative to the observer), the larger it gets and the slower go any and all clocks on it. These facts seem insane and contradict common sense. This is because we have been trained to think that there is only one correct way of explaining things, and everything can be explained in that way. Since we know how nonliving things that we can see or touch work, we believe everything must work in that mechanical way—the way we call "commonsense." We developed this belief in a curious way.

Every science, like every individual, carries within it the marks of its childhood. The common sense of a period in which a science developed becomes the unspoken assumptions of the science. These original assumptions remain within the theoretical framework of the science and strongly influence what will be admissible as real data and what will be automatically rejected as invalid, what will be considered true and what will be considered nonsense. The assumptions will even determine the basic nature of the science's goals and techniques.

Modern science had its childhood in a period when common sense said that the world was made by one God and that He was a rational God. Therefore, the world He created was rational, and there was only one meaning to this term. All things, dreams and machines, the writing of Beethoven's Ninth Symphony, the circling of the planets and the migration of birds, human thought and human feeling, could and must be explained in the same way—within the same system. Long after the idea of the existence of one God was no longer necessarily assumed and accepted, the idea that the whole world could be explained by the same rational system continued to be a fundamental unspoken assumption. Since the assumption was accepted as simply "common sense," it was very difficult to evaluate or test.

Modern science made its first major advances in the sensory realm—those domains of experience in which the data could be seen or touched. The system of rationality that organized the data from this realm had tremendously dramatic and startling results. More progress was made in this realm in 300 years than had been made in the previous 3,000; what was obvious sorcery in 1600 was commonplace by 1900.

In Edgar Allan Poe's "Thousand-and-Second Tale," Scheherezade does not tell the Sultan, as she had in the first thousand and one tales, of Sinbad and Aladdin, of sorcery and magic. Instead, she tells him of the wonders of nineteenth-century science: of the telegraph and the telescope, of the spectroscope and the steam engine. The Sultan responds that always before Scheherezade had told him believable stories, but that this one was preposterous. He then promptly had her executed for having too fanciful an imagination!

If science and its handmaiden, technology, could produce penicillin and washing machines and indoor plumbing, it seemed clear that the laws of science in the sensory realm must be correct. From this it followed that since there was *one* explanatory system for the entire cosmos, this system explained everything that existed—in short, that the system that explained the machine and made it possible to build ever better machines was the only valid system for explaining the rest of reality. Everything that was real would follow the same principles as the machine. Anything that did not follow these principles was not real.

In the sensory world, we know that certain things are true:

1. Everything that is real can be measured and counted (is quantitative in nature).
2. Everything that is real can be taken apart and understood as the sum of its parts.

These two aspects are true of things we can see or touch. They are, generally speaking, true of disease. *They are not true of health.* As we shall see in the next few chapters, one of the obstacles in the way of our understanding "health" is the fact that we have tried to use the common-sense model of reality where it does not apply. The body and physical disease are in the realm of sight and touch, in which this model (and these aspects of it) are valid. Health is in the realm of consciousness, in which they are not.

There are other ways in which the realm of consciousness differs from the realm of experience accessible to the senses—what we loosely term the "see-touch realm." Perhaps the most important difference is that in the see-touch realm there is "public access." More than one person can observe things. Theoretically everyone can see the same things and agree on them. You and I (and, in principle, everyone else) can look at a table and a tape measure and come to the same conclusions about how high and broad the table is. If you tell me it is three feet high and four feet wide, I can check your figures. In the realm of consciousness, however, there is only "private access." Only one person can observe what is going on. This person can report on it to others, but no one can disagree with him. Only I can directly observe my consciousness. Only you can directly observe yours.

The implication of this is that you are the expert—and the only expert—on the subject of your "health." I may serve as a consultant or a guide, but you must make the final observation and decisions.

Thus, in the search for health, each of us must be included as a fully aware participant in the process; we must be informed and we must make decisions. We are the final authority. The specialist working with you in the area of health cannot take a position of authority; he must be a member of a team. The specialist in the area of disease may be able to *tell* you what is wrong with your body. The health specialist can *offer* possibilities for your development and help you to understand your reactions to these ideas.

What has now become clear to us is that a completely unwarranted assumption crept into Western thought over the course of 300 years and became accepted as part of the nature of reality. This assumption was that everything could be understood and explained on the same principles as a machine. Indeed, this is illustrated by the fact that the three most influential systems of thought of the late nineteenth and early twentieth centuries, those of Marx, Darwin, and Freud, all used the machine model. *The evolution of society, the evolution of human beings, and the evolution of the individual personality were all explained on mechanical grounds.* In Marxism, society is seen as a great machine inexorably moving in a certain direction. About the only influence human beings can have on it is to speed up or slow down its progress. In Darwinian theory, evolution takes place according to definite inexorable laws as the accidentally derived characteristics—mutations caused by chance factors (a machine can flip pennies and act on the results)—and ecological possibilities interact. In Freudian theory, the ego is harried and driven by a combination of id drives, superego prohibitions, and cultural possibilities. It must perceive and react to these pressures in strict mechanical fashion, with no room for any such nonsense as free will. The tacit assumption behind all three theories was that any other explanation was false and betrayed a lack of scientific training and information (or, if you did not feel kind—softheaded, muddled, and "medieval" thinking) on the part of the dissenter. One of the greatest of the nineteenth-century scientists, Lord Kelvin, put the common viewpoint clearly when he announced that it was impossible for him to believe in any theory unless he could make a mechanical model of it.

This assumption, and the organization of thought of which it was a part, gave the science of the seventeenth, eighteenth, and nineteenth centuries tremendous power. It brought about the magnificent development of the machine, and our present control of matter and energy. Through the invention of such instruments as the microscope and spectroscope, it opened the way—closed in all previous history—to vaccination, antiseptic and painless surgery, and a host of other boons to the prevention and cure of disease. But in 1900 we began to reach the limit of the mechanistic way of thinking about things. One might legitimately say that the greatest discovery of the seventeenth century (the beginning of modern science) was that one way of explaining things would explain everything in the universe. The greatest discovery of the twentieth century is that it won't.

Because of our history of hundreds of years of belief that there is only *one* true way of explaining the universe and everything in it, any alternative still seems unreal and meaningless. We ask, "But which is the *true* answer, the *correct* system of explanation?" And we expect science to give us a single answer. This, modern science resolutely refuses to do.

The mathematician and theoretician of science Nicholas Rashevsky wrote:

> Half a century ago scientists used to evaluate their theories and theoretical concepts by asking the question: Is the theory or theoretical concept true or false? Since the days of Henri Poincaré, the notion has gradually gained ascendency that the aforementioned criterion is not the proper one. In fact it is not even a meaningful criterion. Nowadays we do not ask whether a given concept is true or false. We ask: Is it convenient or inconvenient; is it useful or not?

If modern science is to continue to advance, we must accept the belief that there is no single answer to the problem of "What is the nature of things." Different answers are needed, ones that are fruitful, and that are valid in different realms of experience. This belief does, it is true, run directly against what we deeply feel to be "common sense": "that collection of prejudices accumulated by age eighteen," as Einstein once defined it. (The philosopher Suzanne Langer defined common sense as ". . . the popular metaphysic of one's generation.") For the fact is that we are still at the beginning of the Planck-Einstein revolution and have only barely begun to understand its implications.

The revolution in science occurred at the same time as similar revolutions were occurring in art. The Impressionists were showing that there was no one correct way to portray reality, but that different concepts of reality were useful for different purposes. Cézanne demonstrated that even in one painting different objects could be depicted as if they were seen from different angles. The artist's eye did not even have to stay in the same place during the painting of a single picture. The use of a variety of concepts of reality and angles of vision has been explored more completely in art during the past century than it has been in science. It is, of course, generally true that in the development of any important understanding, the artist precedes the scientist. The artist makes the intuitive leap to the new comprehension and portrays it in his or her special medium. The scientist (although his progress is also made possible by intuitive leaps such as those of Planck and Einstein) goes more slowly, and only arrives later at the point at which the artist has already arrived.

This is not the place to explore at length the post-Newtonian revolution of thought and its far-reaching implications. For our purposes we need to understand it enough to see how it is effecting changes in medicine today and to appreciate its implications for holistic health practices. As we shall see, one of the great problems in the development of modern science was—and remains—the use of the mechanical, commonsense system of explaining the world in inappropriate realms in which it does not belong. We are just beginning to realize the significance of this problem, and warnings about it are just beginning to appear in the medical literature.

> Each system of concepts can only be legitimately used in the domain of the science to which it belongs. The concepts of physics, chemistry, physiology, and psychology are applicable to the superposed levels of the bodily organization. But the concepts appropriate at one level should not be mingled indiscriminately with those specific of another. For example, the second law of thermodynamics, the law of dissipation of free energy, indispensable at the molecular level, is useless at the psychological level. . . . It is nothing but word play to explain a psychological phenomenon in terms of cell physiology, or of quantum mechanics. . . . Concepts should not be misused. They must be kept in their place. . . .

What does all this mean for our understanding of sickness and health problems? Problems in each realm of experience must be approached with an understanding of the laws and possibilities of that realm. The physician is trained to deal with disease as a problem of the body. Since this is in the see-touch realm, he uses a quantitative and mechanical approach—the correct and *only* method that (with certain qualifications we will come to) can be used successfully. He can use quantitative tests and say a white cell blood count of 3,000 is too low, and one of 16,000 too high. He can separate the various interacting parts of the body and deal first with the blood pressure, and secondarily with the stomach secretion of hydrochloric acid. He can set a bone fracture, and then remove a gallbladder. He thus uses quantitative measures to deal with various body parts and functions, and deals with these separately and in combinations. This is his training: to be a superb mechanic.

"Health," however, is a term primarily applying to the realm of consciousness, the way each person perceives, feels, lives his or her own life experience. In this realm, things cannot be separated from each other. Everything is naturally and organically connected to everything else; there are no "things" at all, only an ongoing process that resumes after interruption by sleep or unconsciousness. "Health" is how we feel and function psychologically. It is predicated on the absence of disease, the correct functioning of the body, but is—in itself—something quite different. For an automobile to work, all the parts—motor, steering wheel, gasoline—must be present and functioning; but for the car to be driven, there must be a driver—a consciousness—behind the wheel.

Health—since it is in the realm of consciousness and meaningful behavior (what we feel, think, and do)—must be approached in ways relevant and valid in these realms. There is no possibility of a quantitative approach to consciousness. My joy can, for example, be stronger today than it was yesterday, but not three times stronger. My pain cannot be quantified as four and a half times as bad as yours. For various reasons, this is an impossibility—despite, I might add, the effort of generations of psychologists to make such quantitative measurements.

Thus the basic orientation of the physician's training, the way he is taught to evaluate and solve problems, is relevant and highly successful in dealing with disease, but simply not applicable in the search for health.

Domain theory is the organization of reality that is the result of the current revolution in scientific thought. According to the theory our experience of the cosmos is divided up into "domains" and "realms." A *domain* is a defined "slice" of reality that we can study in an organized way. All the entities ("observables") we find in it are related to each other by laws. Thus, if we define a domain as a flat, two-dimensional universe, we find it in distances, angles, lines, and shapes (such as squares or circles) and areas, and these are all related by the laws found in the science of plane geometry. If we define our domain as that of the behavior of a large number of interacting particles (such as are to be found in a container of gas), we find pressure, temperature, entropy, and so forth, and we define their relationships through the science of thermodynamics. If we are interested in the domain defined as the interaction of people in a single society, we find the laws governing these interactions through social psychology. In the domain defined as very large bodies of water, the science of oceanography applies.

It is obvious that a very large number of domains can be defined. They can often be redefined to give us different branches of science as our knowledge advances. For example, "psychology" split into a number of domains such as developmental psychology, clinical psychology, social psychology, experimental psychology. Nearly all scientifically defined domains in the past hundred years have undergone similar refinements.

Up to 1900, it was believed (as many scientists and non-scientists still believe) that *all* domains could eventually be understood and dealt with by means of the same system of thought that explained the machine; what was valid in the domains of nonliving things accessible to the senses, it was thought, would be equally so elsewhere. After 1900 we began to understand (and are coming increasingly to understand) that this is not true.

The most profound and least understood concept of the Planck-Einstein revolution was that domains fall into groups called "realms." Each realm comprises all those domains for which the same explanatory system must be used if the data are to make sense. For each realm, therefore, a different way of explaining how reality "works" is necessary.

In different realms the basic "guiding principles," such as "space," "time," "causality," may be different. Thus, in the realm of conscious experience, space is "personal space," not "yardstick space," as it is in the realm accessible to the senses. In this realm, a loved one fifty yards away is "far," an uncaged tiger a hundred yards away is "near," and if we are told that the tiger is hungry, it is "very near." It must be emphasized that these descriptions of space are in no way inferior to the descriptions in yardstick space. They are not less real, they simply apply to different realms of experience. There is a realm of experience, for example, in which space and time cannot be separated, but must be considered as one "space-time." In this realm (that of things that are too large or are whizzing by too fast to be directly accessible to the senses), "space-time" is not an inferior type of description to our usual "space" and "time"; it is not something that will be corrected when we know more; it is the *only* type of spatial description applicable to this realm. The same thing is true of personal space in the realm of consciousness.

Five different realms are now used in science. These are:

1. The realm of the very small.
2. The realm accessible to our senses.
3. The realm of the very large or very fast.
4. The realm of meaningful behavior.
5. The realm of conscious experience.

As we shall see in the following chapters, disease is an observable in the realm accessible to our senses. Once present, it can be dealt with by the use of the mechanical model: the model of reality valid in this realm. Health is an observable in the realm of consciousness. It cannot be dealt with by the mechanical model. Disease and health are not different points on the same continuum; one is not simply an absence of the other. They are entities in two separate realms and—if progress in understanding and control is to be made—they must be approached through different systems of construing reality. For this, in the foreseeable future at any rate, we are going to need two kinds of specialists: the "disease specialist" and the "health specialist."

In the following chapters I shall be describing how this need came about and why it is a basic part of the present development of holistic medicine. I will also describe the types of personality and training necessary to the health specialist, and models of how health specialists and disease specialists can work together. Also I will present material on how to be your own health specialist, and how to design your own unique holistic health programs until such time as the new profession is established and available. At the present rate of change, this should be in the near future.

We are just at the beginning of the Planck-Einstein revolution in which, for the first time, it has been clearly demonstrated that there *are* different realms of experience and these must be dealt with in different terms. Thus we are only starting to realize that selecting and training specialists in disease and selecting and training specialists in health are vastly different matters. There certainly are individuals whose range can encompass both. Most of us are not of this caliber, however. Present developments in medicine indicate that in the future we will have two kinds of training and specialization, one for disease specialists and the other for health specialists. Until that time, however, most of us will have to serve as our own health specialists.

THE APPLICATION OF THE
NEW SCIENTIFIC REVOLUTION
TO MEDICINE

What we have described in the previous chapter is **4**
one of the great revolutions of thought in human history. We might summarize the revolution by saying
that data in each domain of experience must be taken
on their own terms and without preconceptions as to
what they ought to be. The model of the machine on
which nineteenth century science was based, and
which it has been believed would apply to *all* valid
data, is now seen as limited to, and only valid for,
those domains of existence in which things can be—
at least theoretically—seen and touched. In domains
of existence in which things cannot be seen or
touched even theoretically, a different model of reality—a different metaphysical system of explanation—
is needed. To review briefly, a group of domains in
which the data fit a particular model of reality is
called a "realm." At least five different realms, each
needing a different metaphysical system to explain its
particular characteristics, are known to science today:

1. The realm of the too small to see or touch.
2. The realm directly accessible to the senses.
3. The realm of the too large or fast to see or
   touch.
4. The realm of meaningful behavior.
5. The realm of conscious experience.

How does all this apply to the problems of medicine?

The first thing that becomes clear when we apply the new approach—domain theory—to the field of medicine is that sickness and health are domains in two different realms. They are not part of a continuum: they need different kinds of explanatory systems to describe the laws governing their data.

Sickness, the domain physicians are trained and equipped to handle, lies in the see-touch or sensory realm. It is concerned with organs and organ systems and their functioning and breaking down.

Health is a domain in the realms of consciousness and of meaningful behavior. It concerns the ways that human beings potentiate their abilities to be, relate, create, develop. It has to do with the feeling of life and the fullness and color of it. As M. C. Todd, president of the American Medical Association, wrote: ". . . health is not the mere absence of disease, but a positive quality of living."

There are major differences between observables—and the laws relating to them—found in the sensory realm (in which is found the domain of sickness) and the realm of consciousness (in which we find the domain of health). These differences have been described in detail elsewhere and we need only to look at a few of them here.

1. Public versus private access. In the sensory realm, data are public: they may be viewed by any number of people, and if we use scientific methods, all these people will agree as to what they observe. In the realm of consciousness, there is only private access to the data: only one person can view them. He can report to others, and others can examine physiological indicators that tend to accompany certain conscious states (such as blood pressure changes that indicate fear), but only one person can really observe what is going on. One implication of this is that the subject himself is the final judge. If he says, "I feel poorly," or, "I feel well," no one can validly argue with him. Only he

knows if he has a pain in his tooth, although the dentist can evaluate the tooth in the sensory realm. But he has or does not have pain—and if he has, the pain is real—no matter what the X-ray and the dentist report.

This means that in working toward health, the person involved is the only one who can report on how well the process is going, and his word must be taken.

Further, since only one person can be aware of what is going on, what is desirable, what is an acceptable course of action and what is not, the person concerned must be very much a part of the planning process for change. There can be no arbitrary decisions from above as to the best course for this individual: the health specialist can be a consultant, a "guide who knows the landscape," can make suggestions, offer alternatives, point out possibilities, help explore needs and blocks, but the process of designing a program must be one in which the person for whom it is designed is a full partner.

2. Qualitative versus nonqualitative data. The public access data of the sensory realm are quantitative in nature. We can determine that one book weighs two pounds and another weighs three pounds, and know that together they weigh five pounds. All sane men, if equipped with good scales, will agree with this. Data in the realm of consciousness, however, are nonquantifiable in principle. We can say, "I feel happier today than yesterday." We cannot say—and make any sense—"I feel three exuberants of joy today and only felt two and a half yesterday." We can say, "I have a pain," but not "I have three dols of pain." We can say, "I prefer Rembrandt to Magritte," but not "I like Rembrandt four and a half times as much as I like Magritte." Nor can we say that a man who will walk two miles for a Camel cigarette wants a smoke twice as much as a man who will only walk one mile. In the example of the physicist Sir Arthur Eddington, the ponderosity of an elephant is quantitative, but its likableness is not.

E. B. Titchener, who first brought scientific psychology to the United States, wrote in 1896:

> A "thing" is permanent, relatively unchanging, definitely marked off from other things. A process is, by etymology, a "moving forward." It is a *becoming something*—a progressive change which the scientific observer can trace throughout its course. It melts into and blends with operations and changes which follow and precede it. . . . The thing "is" here or there; the process "takes place"—psychology deals always with *processes*, and never with things.

Quantitative measurements turn our view of our data from "processes" into "things." Once we have given a number to something, we undergo a sort of mental compulsion to view that thing as fixed and permanent, rather than as flowing and changing.

We can say of a process that it is moving comparatively slowly or rapidly, smoothly or erratically, in one direction or another, toward a desired or undesired goal, causing pain in its development or the reverse. But it is always a "moving forward" through time.

The health specialist must view the individual person the way Titchener defined a process: as connected to past and future, and blending into them, always flowing and changing.

The implications for the health specialist, once he accepts that his domain is in the realm of consciousness and therefore nonquantitative, are clear. They include the fact that judgments of a life situation must be artistic judgments rather than scientific judgments. We can evaluate a machine quantitatively and say that "three more foot-pounds of force are needed on the end of this lever in order to turn this wheel ten more revolutions per minute." We cannot judge a painting in this way. Rather we can say things like: "This

painting moves me." "It makes me feel good." "I would not
like to have it in my living room." "It affects me strongly."
We are affected or not affected, attracted or repelled, by a
painting. These are artistic judgments, not quantitative ones.

A second difference between domains in the sensory
realm and domains in the realm of consciousness is the lack
in the latter of simple, universal answers to problems. In the
sensory realm, there is a single answer to the problem of
"How long is this table?" or "What is the correct solution to
this mathematical problem?" In the realm of consciousness,
the question "How should a person best live his life?" has as
many answers as there are people. Although we may legitimately place pieces of serious music into categories such as
symphonies, concertos, arias, and so forth, we know that
each piece must be judged as individual and unique; not
compared to others, but only responded to in its own
terms. The same thing is true of paintings, poems, and people. From the health specialist's viewpoint, each person is
unique and must be judged and responded to as such.
There are no "right" answers, but only more or less artistic
answers.

Sickness is thus in a realm where we can deal with states
of existence. It often makes sense to say that an organ is diseased or it is not, a man is sick or he is not. Health is in a
realm where we cannot deal with states, but only with processes. We can say that the flow of a man's development is
distorted, that his aging process is not bringing increased
fulfillment or that it is bringing changing modes of interaction with others.

Aristotle wrote: "The nature of a man is not what he
was born as, but what he was born for." Today we would
say that both are his "nature": what man is "born as" is
in the sickness domain; what he is "born for" is in the
health domain.

The sickness domain contains observables that help us
define how the individual functions in relation to the ques-

tions: "Does he need contact with a medical professional?" "Is there a breakdown of his bodily processes that prevents the potentializing of his capabilities to work, love, enjoy, act, and interact?"

The health domain contains observables that enable us to detect the total pattern of the individual's life. How does he move toward his potential in each period of his existence? How rich and fulfilling is his life? How artistic a pattern is his life making? How richly do his physical, mental, social, and spiritual capacities interact with the possibilities of his culture to form a unique and fulfilling pattern? How much *enjoyment* is there in his life? Is there zest, serenity, gusto, and other qualities in patterns that will fulfill *this* individual's existence and make it worthwhile?

Sickness is essentially defined as a state of deviation from a norm or standard. Therefore, the goal of the sickness therapist is normalcy—normal or average functioning of the body. *Health* is defined as a process leading asymptomatically toward optimal functioning. Therefore the goal of the health therapist is optimal and unique functioning of a particular individual with as little regard for norms or averages as possible.

The sickness domain deals with *"survival"*—how the person survives. The health domain deals with *"thrival"*—how the person thrives.

The sickness domain deals with questions such as "Is anything *wrong* with the functioning of the organism?" These are Abraham Maslow's "D" factors, "deficiency" factors. What is lacking so that progress and positive change cannot occur? Psychotherapy in this realm is the healing of psychological wounds and traumas so that the individual can function in love, and work without pain.

The health domain deals with questions such as "What is *right* with this person? What is his special song to sing, his unique music to beat out in being, relating, creating, transcending?" They are Maslow's "B" factors, "being" factors. Psychotherapy in this realm conforms to the psychiatrist Karen Horney's definition: "A process in which two individuals work together to help one of them take the neurosis, the individuality, from in front of the eyes where it acts as blinders, and move it around to the back of the neck where it acts as an outboard motor."

The sickness domain calls primarily for the approach of the mechanic—to *fix* what is wrong. And since this is a living organism, not a machine, to help the organism fix itself. The sickness specialist—the physician—is an expert in the science of breakdown prevention and repair.

The health domain calls for the approach of the gardener—to help the organism fulfill its potential patterns. In this domain an organism is "well" when it is moving at an optimum rate of development toward its potential for this phase of its existence and weaving all the phases of its life into an artistic whole. The health specialist is—again in Karen Horney's words—"an expert in the art of applying a science that has not yet been invented." (And we would add, since it is an art form, will never be invented.)

The difference between these two approaches is of great importance for the field of medicine. Much of the conflict throughout the history of the healing art has been due to a confusion about these approaches and the uses of each of them. The mechanic is necessary to fix, repair, remove, replace, in situations in which the individual cannot recover from the disease or injury. A perforated ulcer, for example, calls for rapid and expert scientific appraisal and a trained and experienced mechanic to patch the hole and to clear up the resultant infection. Without this, the patient will die, no matter what is done in the way of nutrition, exercise, reorganization of life goals, acupuncture, megavitamins, psychic healers, or changing human relationships. It is only *after* the operation and antibiotics that some of these other activities may become crucial as we strive to understand the *why* of the ulcer. In George Engel's words: "Why did *this*

patient have *this* disease *now*?" We try to understand the ulcer's etiology in order to prevent its reappearance. It is at
this stage that the approach of the gardener is essential. The
gardener, the health specialist, working on the assumption
that disease—or vulnerability to disease—indicates that
something is wrong in the total development, the whole
life, of the individual, examines the pattern, or gestalt, of the
individual's life. His concern is not with damaged or defective organs as such, but with the growth and development
of an entire human being. He asks how this patient is nourishing his body, his mind, and his spirit. Which part of him
is not being nurtured? Which parts of him wait outside the
door of his concern and care? Which parts of him cannot
express themselves? How can this imbalance be corrected?

No matter what the orientation of the health specialist,
one of his first tasks is to see where *this* patient should *start*;
where the first efforts must be made. Should one begin by
reducing the infection, changing the diet, revamping the
life-style? In seeing each patient as an individual, a clear idea
must be formed of the priorities involved. Even the most
devout believers in the efficacy of their particular approach
must be aware of this problem and its crucial nature. St.
Paul (a devout believer, if there ever was one, in the primary nature of the spiritual) wrote: "That is not first which is
spiritual, but that which is natural: then that which is spiritual." (1 Cor. 15:46.)

One holistically oriented internist, Dr. Marvin Meitus, of
Miami Beach, demonstrates this combination in his daily
practice. When a patient comes to see him, he first obtains a
clear picture of the presenting symptoms: why the patient
made the appointment. He then makes a "system review,"
examining and asking questions about each of the major
body organ systems, such as the gastrointestinal system, the
breathing system, the circulatory system. The procedure so
far is quite likely to lead to a diagnosis and to a decision as
to medical intervention. Whether it does or not, however,
Meitus then proceeds—unless there is a medical emergency

present—a further step. He asks the patient to pick a typical day in his life and describe it in detail: what was the first thing done and felt on arising, the second, and so on through the day. In this way, he tries to determine how the patient is functioning in a number of different areas: nutrition, exercise, human relations, creativity, job satisfactions and frustrations, mental stimulation, spiritual activity. If there is specific deficiency in a certain area and Meitus feels it can be handled by simple counseling, he will do so. If he does not feel that such counseling will solve the problem, or if he senses a difficulty but is not able to define it clearly, he will refer the patient to a health specialist, who will then undertake an exploration with the patient of the total pattern of his life. Meitus will continue to supervise the medical aspects of the treatment and such aspects of the total program as nutrition and exercise. He is kept informed of other areas of development. The health specialist, working as would an artist with a painting, tries to understand with the patient in what ways his particular life pattern needs to be changed, expanded, or reorganized to reach its fullest potential, to be most artistically itself.

In the sickness domain a human being is viewed as a closed system within the limits of his skin. In the health domain a human being is viewed as a unique isthmus connecting a particular culture with the universal mind. (Or with those deep archetypical levels of the unconscious where identity merges with the One of existence.)

When we see the patient as a machine, to say, "I do not know what is wrong," reveals our ignorance. When we see him as an organism, it reveals our humanity.

At present, we have great understanding of the sickness domain. We have very little of the health domain. In the words of Reñe Dubos:

We have acquired much information about the body machine and some skill in controlling its responses and correcting its defects. In contrast, we know almost nothing of the processes through which every man converts his innate potentialities into his individuality. Yet, without this knowledge, social and technological innovations are not likely to serve worthwhile human ends.

The specialist in the health domain must take into account the social and spiritual aspects of human beings. These are legitimate observables and influence and interact with observables of the sickness domain. In science, one ignores legitimate observables at one's peril. All the observables in a domain interact and none can be fully understood if the others are not taken into account. Workers in the health domain cannot achieve their ends unless they comprehend the social and spiritual needs and dimensions of humanity.

THE HEALTH SPECIALIST

I plan to explore in this chapter how sickness special- | **5**
ists and health specialists can work together: what is
going on in this developing cooperation and what is
probable for the future. However, before I do this, it
is necessary to look further at this new category of
people—health specialists. What kind of personality
do they need, what kind of training should they ideally receive?

There is a basic philosophy, a point of view, underlying the work of the health specialist. Indeed, it is
a fundamental part of the concept of "holistic
health," which itself is at the center of the changes in
the healing arts that are now under way. This viewpoint has four central aspects.

1. The patient exists on many levels and these are
   of equal importance. He must be considered
   as an individual on *all* of them. In helping the
   person to cure sickness and to approach
   health, we should ideally intervene on as many
   of them as possible at the same time.

   As a corollary of this, there are no such
   things as "alternative modalities of treatment."
   There are "adjunctive" or "complementary modalities of treatment." *Any intelligent and responsible treatment of disease involves the
   care of a physician*. If a health specialist says,
   "Leave all medical treatment and follow my
   path," he is a dangerous charlatan and belongs
   in jail.

2. The patient has self-healing and self-repair systems and these must be regarded as crucial in the prevention and treatment of illness.
3. The patient should be actively and knowledgeably involved in his or her own treatment. The relationship between healer and patient should be one of mutual cooperation between two specialists with special and complementary bonds of information.
4. Each patient is a unique individual and must be met and responded to as such. No person can be validly placed in a classification and then viewed as if the classification contained all that was important about him.

These four principles are the foundation stones of the modern concept of holistic health. It is plain that health specialists will have to have the type of personality and training that will permit them to accept and affirm these ideas *enthusiastically*. Let us take them one at a time.

1. The patient exists on many levels and these are of equal importance.

The poet and philosopher Goethe once wrote, "Nature has neither kernel nor shell." In this aphorism he was expressing the point of view we are discussing. No one level of the individual, no *domain*, is more important than any other. His chemical needs are as crucial as his interpersonal needs (but not more so) and these are as important as his spiritual needs. All are equally real and none can be validly reduced to any other. The health specialist must be a person who understands the fallacy of the "nothing but" idea: that to say that a human being is "nothing but" nine dollars' worth of chemicals is a valid statement only if you plan to use him for fertilizer. Courage is not "nothing but" a reaction formation to passive-dependent needs. Love is not "nothing but" an itching in the groin. A violin concerto is not "nothing but" the dragging of the hairs of a horse's tail over the guts of a cat; religious feeling is not "nothing but" the fear of the dark; and conscious thought is not "nothing but" changing electrochemical states of the brain.

Just as psychology cannot be reduced to biology, so biology cannot be reduced to chemistry. Biological agents, for example, must be tested as such, not as chemical agents. (It is true that we must know their chemistry so that we can reproduce them and standardize them, but they behave quite differently as biological agents than they do as chemical agents.) To demonstrate this, we could use a rather extreme, but valid, example. I take a flask of water that is so chemically pure that no chemical tests will reveal any impurities; none will reveal the presence of anything but water. From a chemical viewpoint it is completely inert. Then I spray it from an airplane over the state of Virginia and destroy the entire tobacco crop of the South. The water contains one molecule of tobacco mosaic virus. Chemically it is inert. Biologically it is a devastating bomb.

Pointing out that each domain must be understood in its own terms and not as a "reduction" of another domain, the psychiatrist Franz Alexander wrote: "It is hardly conceivable that the different moves of two chess players can ever be more clearly understood in biochemical or neurophysiological than in psychological and logical terms."

Eugene Pendergrass, sometime president of the American Cancer Society, has pointed out that the prognosis of cancer patients is very strongly affected by what happens in their personal lives. D. W. Smithers, in England, reported the same experience. Neither of these physicians had had any psychiatric training or experiences. However, they observed and related to their patients, and so saw what the nineteenth-century physician, not separated from his patients by an advanced technology, knew so well. A sizable scientific literature now exists clearly demonstrating the viewpoint of holistic medicine: that the patient exists as a unique and complete person and must be medically evaluated and treated as such, and that all domains of his being interact. In short, that a person, not a group of cells, gets cancer, and that the person, not just his cells, must be evaluated and treated.

What the modern physician frequently forgets is that his actions exist in a context and cannot be meaningfully separated from it. The physician's attitude and beliefs and the patient's conscious and unconscious perception of them strongly affect the results of his medications and procedures. The patient's belief systems about the effectiveness of medical procedures affect how well they work. Since the physician is frequently enthusiastic about new medications, and the patient perceives this, the medications tend to work much better at first than they do later. This is the reason for the old medical adage "Use your new medicine while it still works."

The importance of context is shown in an incident reported by the anthropologist Levy-Bruhl. He tells the story of a South Seas tribe that decided to accept medical treatment from a Western physician. First, however, they decided to accept Christianity, as they could not conceive of the idea that the Christian drugs would work outside of the spiritual setting in which they belonged. This insight is an important one and not to be dismissed lightly as "primitive thinking." Many Western medical procedures of the past (both medical and surgical) were consistently reported by the physicians to produce excellent therapeutic results. They are now considered useless and irrelevant, but at the time, seen as valid by the physician and the patient, they produced many cures. The physicians reporting these results were not fools or dupes. They produced positive results with medical techniques that no longer work because they and their patients believed in the techniques and they pertained to the existing views of reality.

One of the most widely used cures for syphilis in the sixteenth century was guaiacum and there were a great

many attested cures. From the modern point of view, guaiacum is without value in the treatment of syphilis. Nevertheless, there is little doubt that in the sixteenth century it often
was therapeutically effective. This is also true of a great
many other medications and surgical procedures of the
past. We can be certain that in the future, many of our present widely used medications and surgical procedures will
be viewed in the same way.

The importance of the patient's self-healing abilities has
been, perhaps, nowhere shown more clearly than in work
in recent years on the problem of the placebo effect. This
effect has been known for a very long time and it is found
in medical dictionaries as early as 1811. Generally in medicine it has been regarded as a nuisance rather than as a vital
clue to the problems of curing disease. Ignoring it has
slowed medical progress considerably in two ways. First,
the role of the patient's own attitudes and self-repair systems in recovery has been obscured. Second, many medications and surgical procedures have been used and have
worked well until the physician's enthusiasm waned. Excellent reviews of this subject are given in Brian Inglis's *The
Case for Unorthodox Medicine*, and in Jerome Frank's *Persuasion and Healing*. The following paragraphs from Inglis's book may serve as an example.

In the summer of 1962 a report was published of a test
of three drugs used in the treatment of the agonizing
paroxysmal pain known as angina pectoris: iproniazid,
which had been thought to be highly effective, but had
liver damage as occasional side effect; malamide, less
toxic but also presumed to be rather less effective; and
the tranquilizer meprobamate. All three were tested double blind, with placebo controls, and more patients responded better to the placebo than to any of the drugs.
The authors concluded that earlier enthusiastic reports
of improvement based on uncontrolled trials were prob-

ably due "to temporary changes in the mental outlook of the individual patients concerned, or to natural variations in the symptoms."

Such tests bred disillusionment; and it was not only over drugs; if placebo effect was so extensive, physicians countered, might it not be responsible for the "success" of many surgical operations? A great deal of evidence has accumulated to show that this has indeed been the case. In the 1920's, for example, it became fashionable to treat duodenal ulcers by gastroenterostomy; such famous surgeons as W. J. Mayo in the United States and Lord Moynihan in Britain used it extensively. It seemed eminently sensible, since it formed a communication between the stomach and the small intestine, bypassing the pylorus where ulcers originated, "permitting of the discharge of gastric contents into the duodenum, where they belong" (as one enthusiast described it), "and allowing alkaline duodenal contents to pass back into the stomach for the neutralization of gastric acids." Reports were at first almost uniformly gratifying; it was claimed that about 80 percent of patients operated on were still cured five years later, less than two percent suffering from ulcers elsewhere. But eventually a source hostile to the operation reported that the incidence of these "marginal" ulcers following the operation was far higher—in the region of 33 percent; the operation fell out of favor; and it has even been stated that any surgeon using it now would leave himself open to a suit for malpractice.

Since the 1920's, many other forms of treatment of stomach ulcers have been temporarily fashionable; but there is good reason to believe that their successes, too, have been due to placebo effect. In his *Persuasion and Healing*, Dr. Jerome Frank of the Johns Hopkins Hospital, listing many striking examples, included the case of a doctor who experimented on patients with bleeding peptic ulcer, and "70 percent showed excellent results lasting over a period of one year" when the doctor gave them an injection of distilled water, and assured them it was a new medicine that would cure them. A control group, on the other hand, "who received the same injection from a nurse, with the information that it was an experimental medication of undetermined effectiveness showed a remission rate of only 25 percent," which suggests that if the medical profession had been content to exploit suggestion throughout, ulcer patients would have done better during the last fifty years than they have from all the treatments tried—a verdict now gaining official acceptance.

We tend, in our present era, to reduce everything to mechanical models and, in the life sciences, to chemistry. There is the belief somewhere in the back of many of our minds that when science understands enough about chemistry, it will automatically understand biology, then psychology, sociology, and anthropology. Put a different way, many of us have been trained to believe that human thought, feeling, and action can ultimately be *reduced* to chemistry; that chemistry is the *kernel* of life and the rest is *shell*. As we have discussed in chapter 3, this is now an abandoned idea in science, one that needs to be put on the crowded and dusty shelf marked OUTMODED IDEAS—INGEST AT YOUR OWN RISK.

Recently a woman called me for an appointment. She had been diagnosed as having a malignant breast cancer, and surgery and radiation were recommended. She had decided that she wanted nothing more to do with orthodox medicine, and that she would follow an "alternative" path of treatment. Knowing that I specialized in psychotherapy with cancer patients, she had decided to work with me.

During the course of the first hour, after hearing her viewpoint and history, I explained that I conceived of psychotherapy in this type of situation as an attempt to help the patient's cancer defense mechanisms to function more effectively, and to help the patient bring his or her own self-healing and self-repair abilities to the aid of the medical treatment. Psychotherapy with cancer patients is an aid to orthodox medicine, not a replacement.

Toward the end of the hour, we did two things. We phoned and made an appointment for her with Dr. Cushman Haagenson, an extremely experienced and quite conservative oncological surgeon at Columbia Presbyterian Hospital. We also set up a series of appointments for psychotherapy.

Some time later, another cancer patient phoned me for an appointment. He had been referred to me by a surgeon in Chicago. He had had three cancer primaries (an almost unheard-of event) in two years and had had several metastases from one of them. The viewpoint of his oncologist was that his cancer defense mechanism was in almost total collapse. During the course of the first hour, we arranged the timing for regular psychotherapy sessions and also made an appointment for him with the Craig Institute in Holbrook, Long Island, which specializes in nutritional programs in severe illness.

With both of these patients, as the exploration of their lives progressed, we tried to comprehend together their interpersonal needs, their creative possibilities, the unique *context* of their lives. We learned to see for each the gestalt, or pattern, of their physical, psychological, and spiritual being. As William James understood so well: "There is no valid demarcation between philosophy and physiological psychology."

The health specialist must *know* that each level of a human being, each domain of his existence, is equally valid and interacts in a fluid way with all of the others. He must not be so ill at ease with, or afraid of, the larger aspects of his own life—his feelings, his creativity, his social and his spiritual needs—that he attempts to *reduce* them, to say that they are "nothing but" unconscious psychodynamics, reinforced chains of reflexes, or chemical interactions. He must be fully able to accept, celebrate, and nurture these parts of himself so that he can do the same with his patients.

I cannot overemphasize how important it is that health specialists should be knowledgeable in an approach to the human condition other than that taught in a social science department or in a psychiatric setting. The training in psychology and psychiatry is much more narrow than is generally understood and certainly more narrow than is realized by most of the graduates. In this training, one is likely to learn a great deal about unconscious personality dynamics, ego defenses, Oedipal problems, dependency, and sibling rivalry. One may even learn about social class personality interactions, drug addiction, and Korsakow's psychosis. It is extremely unlikely that one will be taught anything about responsibility, dignity, courage, compassion, sadness, strength in adversity, or love. For these one must go elsewhere—to the arts and the humanities. Here the best and wisest of our race have been struggling for all of history to understand and express our pain and joy, our foolishness and wisdom, our narrowness and greatness.

> Placed on this isthmus of a middle state,
> A being darkly wise, and rudely great;
> With too much knowledge for the Sceptic side,
> With too much weakness for the Stoic's pride,
> He hangs between; in doubt to act, or rest;
> In doubt to deem himself a God, or Beast;
> In doubt his Mind or Body to prefer;
> Born but to die, and reas'ning but to err; . . .
> Created half to rise, and half to fall;
> Great lord of all things, yet a prey to all;
> Sole judge of Truth, in endless Error hurl'd;
> The glory, jest, and riddle of the world!
>   —ALEXANDER POPE

In the textbooks and seminars of psychiatric, psychological, and social-work training, these aspects of being human are as little discussed as is the field of nutrition in most medical schools. One must go elsewhere to learn about them.

> ... solving problems of disease is not the same thing as creating health and happiness. This task demands a kind of wisdom and vision which transcends specialized knowledge of remedies and treatments.
>
> —RENÉ DUBOS

After Martha Gassman had been my control (or training) therapist for a year or so, she looked at me one day and said: "Larry, it's about time we started getting you educated." I muttered angrily about a Ph.D. from the University of Chicago being an indication of *something*. She replied that I indeed did know a great deal about ego defenses, nomenclature, and the different schools of psychotherapy. She went on, "You're a pretty good *mechanic*, and in time you will become an excellent one. You know most of what is important in the textbooks of psychology and psychiatry. But in the fields that work with what it means to be human, you are an ignoramus. You know nothing about music, art, literature, classics, or philosophy. You do know and love poetry and that's a healthy start. But if you want to be more than a mechanic, if you want to be a *therapist*, you have a lot of work and growing to do. Here is a first reading list." I still have that list. It includes *Paradise Lost*, *The Republic*, some Carlyle. There was also a list of museums to visit. Presently, of course, I found areas that appealed to me and studied on my own. I have much to thank Martha Gassman for, including the fact that I believe I am still struggling on the road to becoming a *therapist*.

The psychiatrist Kurt Goldstein wrote: "When a student of human nature bases his studies on the result of one special science, he has nothing but a starting point; he will never derive a correct answer to his questions from the material of a single realm alone."

One must, in selecting health specialists, beware of the

person who is educated far beyond his or her intelligence. As the philosopher Chuang-Tse wrote in 400 B.C., "With a learned person it is impossible to discuss the problems of life; he is too bound by his system." The person who is full of facts, able to quote all sorts of references and experiments, but who brings no larger viewpoint, no share of wisdom and its handmaiden, gentleness, to bear, may well be a mechanic, but cannot be a gardener. Further, he is likely to go to quite ridiculous extremes as long as he views everything through the narrow lenses of a particular system, forgetting that life is far too rich, colorful, and charged with meaning and feeling ever to be encompassed in a single system. The British philosopher C. D. Broad once described behaviorism (which tries to explain all the scope of being human on the basis of reflexes), as "one of those systems so innately silly that they could only have been devised by very learned men."

The viewpoint of the gardener, quite opposite to this, is illustrated in the following story. Some years ago, the child psychiatrist Annina Brandt was speaking to the professional staff of a Westchester child-guidance clinic. The staff of this clinic was, at this time, very psychoanalytically oriented and saw all behavior in terms of this particular system. As Brandt talked in her loving way of children, revealing the scope, intensity, and variety of their inner worlds, the staff became more and more uncomfortable and restless. Finally one of them broke in and asked, "Dr. Brandt, what *school* do you belong to?" Brandt looked startled, thought a bit, and then said in a puzzled way, "But how can I tell until I see the child?"

Kenneth Walker in his *Doctors and Patients* wrote:

The disadvantages of specialization are as obvious as are its advantages, and they have been crystallized in the popular saying that a specialist is "a man who knows more and more about less and less." In other words, the specialist is a man who takes a very lop-sided view of his patient, seeing him only through the tiny peephole of his own specialty. To the ear, nose, and throat expert, a patient is not so much a person as a supporting structure for infected tonsils, poorly drained sinuses, middle ear disease, and laryngeal troubles, and to the dermatologist he is little more than a perambulating background to interesting rashes. Even when specialists work together as a team, as they do in hospitals and well-organized clinics, they must begin by taking their patient to pieces, and they do this so effectually that he may never be seen again as a complete person. During his passage through the various departments of the clinic, his *dossier* collects an immense amount of interesting notes, graphs, X-rays, and chemical, pathological, and bacteriological reports, but less and less is known about him as a human being.

. . . We are far more "fearfully and wonderfully made" than even the Old Testament writer of these words was aware. And just as something is much more likely to go wrong with the working of an extremely intricate instrument than with the working of a simple one, so are we highly differentiated human beings more liable to become ill than are such simple kinds of organisms as amoebae, turnips and jelly-fish. We are capable of experiencing harmonies and discords within our complex being of which these simple creatures know nothing, and to be accounted truly healthy we must attain harmony not on one but on three planes—the physical, the psychological, and the spiritual. These three entities or qualities within us are so closely interwoven as to be inseparable, so that a disturbance in one of them is communicated quickly to the others.

"The uncharted surrounds us on every side, and we must needs have some relation to it. . . ." wrote the classicist Gilbert Murray. Carl Jung observed on the basis of many years of experience with patients from all over the world, that he had never seen a patient over thirty-five whose problem was not in essence a religious problem, and no cure of the illness could be achieved until the religious problem was cured. Jung here was not speaking of church membership or attendance. (Too often the established religious organizations act—in philosopher Walter Huston Clark's analogy—like a vaccination: they give us a small case of the disease in order to prevent us from getting a larger one.) Jung was speaking of the problem of the meaning of one's life—of the *context* within which one acted and lived. Until we are able to establish a harmony between our inner nature, the specific structure of our individual being, and the needs of our species as a part of the general nature of the cosmos, we tend to become ill and we maintain this tendency until we attune our life and actions to this larger context.

2. The patient has self-healing and self-repair systems and these must be regarded as crucial in the prevention and cure of illness.

In the first chapters of this book, I have written about the age-old conflict in the healing arts as to whether the practitioner primarily should actively *intervene* with strong methods such as surgical and chemical procedures, or primarily should *cooperate* with the self-healing abilities of the patient. The battle between these two viewpoints has gone back and forth, and each historical period has leaned toward one or the other. Today we are realizing that we need both. The major communicable and infectious diseases have largely been conquered by the advances in intervention medicine; the degenerative diseases have not. Nor have advances in surgical and chemical methods given us clues as to differences in susceptibility and to recovery rates. They have taught us much about disease, little about health. Further, they have led to strong and growing discontent with modern medicine on the part of the general public. We are at the end of a period in which intervention medicine has been the guiding philosophy in medical training and practice, and in which the importance of the patient's self-restitutive system has been generally overlooked.

As we have said before, the present trend is not toward the other extreme; the pendulum has, to a great extent, stopped swinging. Instead of continuing with our usual "either-or" approach, we are moving toward a "both-and" viewpoint.

The health specialist must be a person who can recognize and emotionally accept that his work with the patient is invaluable, but only as part of a larger whole that includes the work of the sickness specialist in equal partnership. If he is competitive, if he is on a power trip, his influence will be destructive, not constructive. He will be unable to work with the physician who is in the role of disease specialist, and will also be unable to work with the patient. Helping the patient find his own unique blend of life activities is vastly different from finding it for him. It is one thing to give a hungry person a fish, it is another to teach him the art of fishing. The health specialist must be a person who can work not only with disease specialists, but also with the patient as an equal partner. He must be comfortable with the role of guide and companion in the search, and not feel emotionally compelled to be superior. "The real guru," the mystic Pir Vilayet Khan said, "is one who kills the idol you have made of him."

Many years ago I was fortunate enough to be taught psychotherapy by the psychiatrist Abraham Meyerson. One day he looked long and searchingly at each of the eight of us in the class and said, "In your work, you will often be tempted to play God." He paused a long moment and then added, "And so few of you have the qualifications." He then walked out of the room and shut the door behind him, leaving us silent as each of us reviewed our own qualifications and found them sadly lacking. In a few minutes the door opened again; Meyerson put his head in and added, "And besides, the job is taken!"

In his work, the health specialist cannot play God. Only by helping the patient find his own unique path and his own special pattern of growth can the health specialist help the patient mobilize his life forces and move toward health. He does this as one who cooperates with the patient's own healthy forces, not as one who knows the goal, plans the program, and directs each step. He is a facilitator, not a major general.

The historian Jacob Bronowski wrote:

> Man masters nature not by force but by understanding
> . . . in four hundred years since the Scientific Revolution,
> we have learned that we gain our ends only *with* the
> laws of nature. . . .We cannot even bully nature by any
> insistence that our work shall be designed to give power
> over her. We must be content that power is the byprod-
> uct of understanding. So the Greeks said that Orpheus
> played the lyre with such sympathy that wild beasts
> were tamed by the hand on the strings. They did not
> suggest that he got his gift by setting out to be a lion
> tamer.

3. The patient should be actively and knowledgeably involved in his/her own treatment.

One patient with a long-term illness put it, "Every doctor I've ever met had more confidence in his evaluation of
my condition than in my evaluation of my condition."

A study of the present medical situation by Thomas
Szasz and Marc H. Hollander described three main models
of physician-patient interaction: "activity-passivity," "guidance-cooperation," and "mutual interaction." In activity-
passivity relationships, the patient is completely passive, as
in surgery, electroconvulsive shock, or forced drugging in
schools or prisons. In guidance-cooperation relationships

the patient suffers and seeks help. He places the physician in a position of power, and the physician initiates most of the action. The patient is expected to do what he is told.

In mutual participation relationships, the " . . . physician does not profess to know exactly what is best for the patient. The search for this becomes the essence of the therapeutic interaction. . . ." Initiation of interaction is more or less equal. The patient essentially manages a good deal of the process himself.

It is this third type of interaction that would be found in work with a health therapist. All three kinds (with the emphasis, ideally, on the last) would be found in working with a therapist in the sickness domain.

> The patient has to participate in his own treatment. He must *help himself* to get well. Participation is more than taking a pill every day. He must choose a diet, exercise, relaxation, etc. Pretty soon you get patients who are no longer taking pills. . . . The miracle cure is when the patient helped cure himself. . . . It's more important what you don't do for a patient than what you do. . . . When a patient says, "What can I do to help?" you are in a new ball game.
>
> —M. MEITUS, M.D.

The importance of patient participation in medical procedures is shown in the present acceptance of the "natural childbirth" movement, and the role of the modern midwife. One of the most appealing aspects is that it allows the mother—and where possible the father and often the whole family—to be a full and educated part of the birth process. The entire experience of birth is changed by a good midwife from a "thing" that is happening to the mother's body, and toward which she is passive (except for exhortations to "push") to an integral part of the entire fabric of life in which the mother and father are active participants. A seri-

ous midwife has a good comprehension of the basic axioms
of holistic medicine. She sees the birth preparation and
process as one part of the total symphony of the family's life
and tries to help the family see them in this way. She is constantly aware that the mother exists in many equally important domains, and is sensitive to, and refers to, specialists in
nutrition, vitamin usage, exercise, psychotherapy, relationship needs, and spiritual concerns. She sees each patient as
an individual who must be assessed, treated, and responded
to as unique, and not as a member of a class of clients. She
establishes a relationship with her clients as an equal rather
than as an authority figure who acts out "mother knows
best." Being a responsible practitioner of adjunctive medicine, she also works with medical supervision and emergency backup.

As we have seen earlier in this chapter, if the health specialist wishes to help the patient move toward health, the
patient must be involved as an active and equal partner.
There are no *right* roads toward health, but only a best road
for each individual. Since health is an observable in the
realm of consciousness, and in this realm there is only private access—only one person, the patient himself, can observe the data—the patient is as expert as the therapist. The
patient knows the *ground* of his life, its color and texture,
better than anyone else can. The therapist has a wider view
and is more knowledgeable and experienced in many of the
problems relating to health. Working together, they can
form an effective and smoothly functioning team, but only
the patient can judge how he feels or determine whether a
procedure is helping or not. He alone is in the *midst* of his
life and experiences it directly. Even gifted with the greatest
possible empathy, the therapist is at a distance. In Goethe's
words, "Gray are all your theories, but green the growing
tree of life."

It is this respect for the patient, as a person and as the
only real expert in how his own life is and feels, that is es-

sential for the health specialist. If he cannot achieve this stance—as many cannot—he does not have the personality structure that will enable him to understand holistic medicine or to function in it.

If a physician or other health provider is younger than you are and addresses you by your first name early in your relationship, beware! We prefer younger strangers—even if they are physicians—to address us as Miss, Ms., Mrs., or Mr. Doing so shows respect for us and not doing so shows quite the opposite. (I have known twenty-five-year-old interns to call older women "Mary" at their first meeting and have generally decided that the intern is probably not educable.)

> 4. Each patient is a unique individual and must be met and responded to as such.

> If you give the same nutrient to a patient with a fever and to a person in health, the patient's disease is aggravated by what adds strength to the healthy man.
>
> —HIPPOCRATES

Hans Selye, who first developed the modern concept of "stress," presents three guidelines in *Stress Without Distress* for living fully amid the "wear and tear of everyday life," without illness or disease. The first of these guidelines is: "Find your own natural predilections and stress *level*. . . . Only through planned self-analysis can we establish what we really want; too many people suffer all their lives because they are too conservative to risk a radical change and break with tradition."

Today we are beginning to understand that individualized treatment programs, tailored for the person involved, are crucial for all the arts of medicine and healing. Anyone—nutritionist, physician, chiropractor, psychotherapist, psychic healer—who does not comprehend this, should be avoided like the plague he is.

The great teachers of mysticism have always understood

that in psychic and spiritual development, there is a different path for each person.

In her autobiography, St. Thérèse of Lisieux wrote of the problems of being a spiritual director:

> I know it seems easy to help souls, to make them love God above all, and to mold them according to His will. But actually, without His help it is easier to make the sun shine at night. One must banish one's own special tastes and personal ideas and guide souls along the special way Jesus indicates for them rather than along one's own particular way.

When the Seer of Lublin was asked to name one general way to the service of God, he replied: "It is impossible to tell men the way they should take. For one way to serve God is through learning, another through prayer, another through fasting, and still another through eating. Everyone should carefully observe what way his heart draws him to, and then choose this way with all his strength."

In a similar vein, Rabbi Nachman of Bratislava wrote: "God calls one man with a shout, one with a song, one with a whisper."

I recall a wise and expert psychoanalyst (Dr. Joseph Michaels) saying to a hospital psychiatric service staff conference, "I am prescribing the SNARIB treatment for this patient. It will do him far more good than psychotherapy or than anything else in the pharmacy." He then turned to the physician who had presented the case and, asking him to make sure that the treatment was carried out, left the conference room. Each of us, not having the faintest idea what this method consisted of, resolved to look it up immediately. When a library search failed to turn up a reference to a SNARIB treatment or even to a Dr. Snarib, we went back to Michaels in a group and asked him what he had been referring to. He told us that the term was an acronym for the one method that our medical and psychotherapeutic training had not prepared us for. It stood for "Skillful Neglect and Rest in Bed." Michaels then continued, "This is what *this* patient needs. He is a completely typical patient in that he is unique and what he needs is unique. Anytime you find two patients who need exactly the same treatment, you can be sure that the similarity is in your perception of them, not in them. And if you see more than two who need the identical treatment, it is quite likely that you are perceiving your own problem, not theirs, and prescribing for them what should be prescribed for you."

It is hard to overemphasize the importance of this point. So accustomed are we to believing that there is one right way to do things that doctors tend automatically to slip into treating patients according to this concept. The belief is strengthened by long years of medical education that emphasizes one cause for each disease and one correct procedure to follow in combating it.

We differ tremendously from each other in our genetic heritage, in our childhood and adult experience of the world, in the degree and ways that we have nurtured or repressed our different needs, in the amount and ways we have directed our energies inward and outward, in our fears of ourselves and others, and in the meaning we have found for our lives. Knowledge of these differences is not just of theoretical interest, but is crucial for work at all levels of the treatment of disease and the search for health. One reason a trained anesthesiologist is required at every major surgical procedure is that each person differs in his response to an anesthetic and an expert is required to monitor the patient throughout the operation. A responsible physician who decides to prescribe a tranquilizer or other mind-influencing drug will not choose the most popular one in the general classification desirable, but will hand-tailor the prescription to the particular patient, and then will evaluate the patient's response at frequent intervals to see how this unique individual tolerates the medication. He knows that no two people respond to any chemical intervention the same way.

Abraham Meyerson used to say, "As soon as you have decided, on the basis of theory and experience, that all patients who have 'A' also have 'B,' and that this can be absolutely depended on, you can be absolutely certain that within three days, a patient will come into your office with 'A' and not the slightest sign of 'B.' This will happen. The only question is will you be too blind to see it?"

Unfortunately a large percentage of disease specialists and practitioners of adjunctive modalities are chronically blind in this direction. They are so certain of their theory and experience that they are unable to notice individual differences. This inability kills a lot of people.

A few years ago I brought a close relative to Mt. Sinai Hospital in New York City (a large teaching hospital with an excellent reputation) for major abdominal surgery. The drug of choice at the hospital for pain control during recovery was Demerol. This particular person did not respond to Demerol; for her it had no more effect than a sugar pill. I made sure that I told this both to the surgeon and the anesthesiologist. For good measure (I *am* experienced with hospital rigidity) I saw that on her chart in large red letters was written "allergic to Demerol." (There are, by the way, a number of excellent and equally effective morphine-based drugs for pain control such as Dilaudid, Pantopon, or morphine itself.) After the surgery, in the recovery room, she was, of course, given a large dose of Demerol. She was eventually brought back to her hospital room on a stretcher, screaming in pain and with blood pressure and temperature dangerously below normal and dropping. Since she had had a large dose of Demerol, nothing more could be given to her for some hours. The chief resident was called and was understandably concerned. He hovered in attendance, doing his best until the absolute minimum time was up. He then went to the floor's nursing station and came back with a loaded hypodermic which he immediately injected into her. When after five minutes it had no effect, I asked him what it was. He replied, with surprise at my question, that of course it was Demerol, what they always used for severe postsurgical pain. This meant that she had to go through another three hours without pain relief, during which time she very nearly died. But for the happy fact that a couple of Delores Krieger's* expert and holistically trained nurses had come by to see how she was doing, she would have. These nurses were able to get the patient through the next few hours of pain and raise her blood pressure and temperature by the use of breathing and movement exercises, meditation, autohypnosis, and psychic healing. They saved her life, but a basic flexibility of mind and openness to new experience (not to mention an attention to the patient's medical chart) on the part of the medical staff would have obviated the crisis in the first place.

For the health specialist, no two people can be treated the same. This is the reason that the only universally valid law in psychotherapy is Miale's Law, which states that "any response which comes from technique rather than human feeling is antitherapeutic." *Technique* refers to a stereotyped way of responding to *classifications* of people. If we treat people as if what is important about them is *only* the classification we have given them, we reduce them to less than they are, and so our response is antitherapeutic. The pattern of each person's life, and its possibility for expansion, is as different for each person as it is for each serious painting or piece of music.

One of the great Hassidic rabbis, Shneur Zalman, was in prison and was being examined about his beliefs. During the examination, he was asked, "What do you understand by the scriptural words that God, the All-Knowing, said to Adam, 'Where art thou?'" The rabbi answered that the Scriptures are eternal and every era, every generation, is in-

---

*Delores Krieger is a professor of nursing at New York University Graduate School. She trains her nurses in an unusually holistic approach to the patient at all levels of being from the chemical to the psychic.

cluded in them. "In every era, God calls out to man: 'Where are you in your world? So many years and days of those allotted to you have passed and how far have you gotten in your world?' God says something like this: 'You have lived forty-six years. How far along are you?'"

The health specialist will be developing individuals who are resistant to tyrannical governments and fascist philosophies of both the left and the right. Able to account to themselves for their lives and to be autonomous, they will not be likely to seek refuge from their anxiety in passively accepting a dogma. As the serious artist examines and then rejects the artistic fads of the moment, these artistic creators of their own lives will resist the mass explanations and directives of real and would-be dictators. The more a person is an individual, the less he fits in a mass movement, and the goal of the health specialist is the individualizing of life.

The health specialist must always be aware that the pattern of *this* patient's life is a unique and organic whole. What is truly good for one part is good for the whole and vice versa. For the gardener there is a proper goal for each plant—the fullest blooming as itself. The root, the stalk, and the blossom are integral and essential parts of the completely individual whole.

One of the most impressive developments in the evolution of holistic health has been the development of the hospice movement, started by Cicely Saunders in England during the 1960s. Saunders observed from her experience as a nurse that hospitals were ill equipped to deal with the needs of the dying patient. She envisioned a new type of institution that would fill these needs.

In order to actualize her dream, she took further training and gained degrees in social work and medicine. She then opened the first hospice in London. St. Christopher's Hospice was a hospital especially suited to the dying person.

Today there are a large and growing number of hospices in England and the United States. They are staffed with trained people who are not afraid to relate to the dying person as an individual. They are able to discuss with the patient anything he wishes to and are not constrained by their anxiety to reassure constantly or change the subject and talk about the weather when the patient brings up questions about life and death, living and dying, sadness, pain, or any of the other large questions we generally manage to avoid until forced to face them by the great events of our lives.

One patient, dying of cancer of the lymphatic system, said to me: "You know, Larry, most of us never face the big questions of life. But once you pick them up, you can't put them down until you have found an answer for you." An approaching death raises these questions, but it is generally made perfectly clear to the dying patient that no one in the family or the hospital will discuss them or help the patient to face them. Doctors, nurses, family members, and, sadly enough, even most hospital chaplains reassure, offer clichés, and quickly find they are needed elsewhere if the patient talks about them. Treated like a child, unable to discuss the things most on his mind, surrounded by a conspiracy of silence, the patient is frequently like Tolstoi's dying Ivan Ilych. "In the bosom of his family, he was more alone than if he had been at the bottom of the sea or on the other side of the moon."

The psychiatrist Carl Jung told of the following incident: Because of a change in her husband's job, one of his patients was forced to discontinue the analysis and leave the city. One day, he received a call from a local hospital. They told him that they had a dying patient who had become psychotic. A relative had told the hospital that many years before she had been a patient of Jung's. Would he come to see her and try to help them understand why she had become psychotic?

Jung looked up her records and went to the hospital. He found the woman in bed, very ill, and talking to herself. At first he could not understand what was going on. What she was saying seemed completely irrelevant to the hospital situation. As he sat and listened, however, it suddenly dawned on him that she was finishing the analysis that she had had to terminate so many years before. He sat, fascinated, by her bedside for several weeks while she completed the work of analysis, finding out who she was and the meaning of her life. After she was done she seemed very tranquil and died peacefully.

I have written earlier of human spiritual needs. The need to make sense out of our existence is a deep and important drive within us. Few of us are like Jung's patient, who could, of necessity, undertake the process alone. As holistic medicine, with its emphasis on the validity of a person's needs and the necessity of integrating a life into one artistic creation, continues to develop, there will be increasing numbers of therapists who can help the dying patient perceive the meaning that he could not perceive earlier.

Hospices are run by holistically oriented professionals and lay persons who see and relate to the dying person as a complete person whose approaching death is part of the total fabric of his life. They see their task as one of making this last period as meaningful and enriching as possible and of helping the patients find the significance and values of their lives. (As one patient put it to me, the hospice staff had helped him "find out what my own name is and how much I lived under it and how much I didn't and the reasons why.") Some of the hospices have their own buildings, as does St. Christopher's. Some operate within a hospital. Some are organized "without walls" and operate in the community. Exemplifying the best of this last type is Charles Garfield's beautifully managed Shanti Project in San Francisco. In Garfield's training program, lay people learn how to do hospice work. They find that it is not only their patients whose lives are enriched and given meaning, but also their own.

The holistic health movement is developing in so many ways and its influence has spread in so many directions throughout our medical system that it is impossible to describe them all. One noteworthy area, however, is the work done over the last few years in refugee camps.

This work started in 1979 when an unusually well-trained San Francisco health specialist, Dr. Virginia Veach, became concerned about the reports reaching the United States of the conditions in the Cambodian refugee camps on the border of Cambodia and Thailand. She began organizing holistic medical teams of ten to twelve persons each, consisting of physicians, nurses, physical therapists, paramedics, psychologists, and laboratory technicians. Each team (there were five of them) in rotation would take over a ward of approximately one hundred patients in a camp hospital. The teams stayed in Cambodia from two to six months.

The team members, in addition to mainline medical abilities, brought a variety of skills to bear. For example, when patients are malnourished past a certain point and the body begins digesting its own protein (muscles and cartilage), many standard medications are no longer effective. The body's chemistry has changed so much that antibiotics, quinine, and a variety of other medicaments simply no longer work. The Veach teams found that starving patients could be brought back to a condition of responsiveness to these substances if someone simply stayed with them for a few days, bringing up the body's water supplies by spoon feeding, stroking, touching, and psychic healing. They found, in Veach's words, that "there is a real difference between a spoonful of water put into a patient's mouth impersonally and a spoonful put into the mouth by someone who cares and is 'with' the patient." (It is now generally accepted in medicine that in intensive care units a good deal of touching and handling of the patients, under any loving pretext, enables them to do much better and recover much faster than when this is not done.) The people on the holistic teams were trained in local religious beliefs and taboos and in fundamental respect for their patients as individuals. The results more than justified the work.

There was a markedly lower death rate in the holistic medicine ward than in the wards staffed by first-class mainstream medical teams from all over the world. The medical coordinator of Camp Khao I Dang (where the teams operated) stated that the most difficult cases in the hospital were referred to the holistic ward and that "the recovery rate, by all standards, medical as well as psychological, was remarkable." In spite of some initial reservations, the hospital director was enthusiastic about the teams' work and has written letters in their support to the International Catholic Migration Commission—the sponsoring organization. It is of interest that all personnel were volunteers and that not only were all of them unpaid, but all organizing was done on Veach's own time and, except for telephone charges, at her own expense.

St. Thomas Aquinas wrote in the *Summa*: "We do not offend God except by doing something contrary to our own good." There can be no contradiction between our caring for the physical and the emotional and spiritual elements of our being. As Aquinas knew so well, what is truly good for one of these elements of the gestalt that is our being is in essence positive for the others. "God exercises care over every person on the basis of what is good for him. Now it is good for each person to attain this end, whereas it is bad for him to swerve away from his proper end."

As we have shown, the health specialist must have a personality and training that allow him to work smoothly within the four basic axioms of holistic medicine. What else can we say about his necessary qualifications?

Certainly he must be well trained and experienced in his particular specialization. As Maimonides wrote:

The more perfect a person becomes in one of the sciences, the more cautious he grows, developing doubts, questions and problems that are only partially solved.

And the more deficient one is in science, the easier it will be for him to understand every difficulty, making the improbable probable and increasing the false claims which he represents as certain knowledge, and eager to explain things that he does not understand himself.

The personality qualifications we have discussed, plus good will, are not enough. A nutritionist must *know* a great deal about nutrition, and this knowledge can only be achieved by hard work and study. Reading *Prevention* magazine and popular books on the subject and being a vegetarian is not enough. Similarly a psychotherapist must have intensively studied Sigmund Freud, Carl Jung, Alfred Adler, Karen Horney, Kurt Goldstein, Andras Angyal, Viktor Frankl, Abraham Maslow, and others, have had effective psychotherapy himself, and years of supervision. There is no substitute for hard work and supervised experience in any of the health specialties. But assuming this professional competence, what else is needed?

In the same way that we would not go to a gymnastic instructor who had a soft and flabby body, we would expect a specialist in the health domain to reveal through his own life that he or she comprehends the meaning of health. The therapist should exhibit appropriate signs of serenity, zest, joy. He should have a concern for his own physical, mental, social, and spiritual well-being and for how the needs and relationships of these change in different periods of his life.

The therapist will need to have positive relationships with himself, others, and the natural world of which we are all a part. (I am reminded here of the Test for Spiritual Advancement humorously devised by the San Francisco psychiatrist Arthur Deikman. It is to be used for evaluating a potential "guru" and has but one deadly question: "How does he get along with his wife?" Clearly Deikman is not concerned in this test only with marital relationships, but with all human relationships.)

Further, we would expect this person to be actively *working* on his own growth and development. Anyone who says that he has arrived at his goals in life reveals only that he has extremely limited goals. One never "gets there," one only works toward growth. As Gertrude Stein once put it: "When you get there, you find there is no there there"; or, in Abraham Maslow's words: "Self-actualization is not a static, unreal perfect state in which all human problems are transcended, and in which people 'live happily ever after' in a superhuman state of serenity or ecstasy."

Unless a person can actively tend to himself, he cannot tend to others. One cannot validly say, "Do as I say, not as I do." Unless he can grow and change himself and work at it, he cannot signal others to do the same. The health specialist must be able to grow and learn. He must be an individual who, after twenty years of work experience, has had twenty years of experience, and not someone who has one year of experience repeated twenty times.

In order to be a health specialist, one must be a caring person. One of the rare oncologists who works in both the domain of sickness and the domain of health—Laurens White of San Francisco—said at a medical conference: "Our patients do not demand that we cure them. They demand that we care for them." In his classic paper of 1927, Francis Peabody wrote: "The secret of the care of the patient is in caring for the patient."

Certainly the behavior of the health specialist must imply a set of values. Rather than trying to present these in abstract terms, let us try to give a specific example. Let us each imagine a person of the sort that we admire, a mature person who acts out our values and lives in the way we wish the whole world would live. Further, let us imagine that this person knows us deeply and well and loves and cares about us in the way that a "good" parent, teacher, or psychotherapist cares. He or she truly wants the best for us. Now let us ask: What would this person want for us? What would he or she *choose* for us? As Maslow has pointed out, the healthier and more mature a person is, the better *chooser* he is. What this person would choose for us would reveal the values that ideally should underlie and organize the behavior of the health specialist. For each of us the choice would be unique. For each of us the choice would potentiate our lives, including our relationships with others. The choice would direct each of us toward a life that would fulfill our unique and species-wide inner nature. But until we possess the kind of health specialists we are imagining, we can work toward becoming our own health specialist by learning to make choices that the "good" parent would make for ourselves. Often, a psychotherapist can aid us in learning how to understand and love ourselves.

The most widely used adjunctive modality today is psychotherapy. The relationship with the practitioner is potentially the most personal, involved, and close of all the modalities. It is therefore necessary to say a few special words about choosing a psychotherapist. What I say here also applies, but to a somewhat lesser degree, to choosing any practitioner, including a physician.

As always, professional competence comes first. The therapist must be a psychiatrist, a psychologist, or a social worker. If a psychiatrist, he or she should be Board certified or Board eligible and a member of the American Psychiatric Association. If a psychologist, he should have at least a master's degree and be a member of the American Psychological Association. A social worker should have a master's degree and membership in the National Association of Social Workers. The best way to find qualified people is by referral from a professional you trust and/or by asking the state or city branches of the organizations mentioned. Recommendations from friends are frequently useful.

But professional training and competence, although essential, are not enough. There are other requirements. First, it is important that you *like* the therapist. If you don't, you may be able to make progress with him or her, but it will take you at least nine times as long and be nine times as difficult. A therapist is not a mechanic adjusting you to work better; a therapist is a guide and companion on a hard but exciting road. Unless the chemistry is right between you, unless there is an intuitive rapport, the road will be much harder.

At the end of the first session, ask yourself some questions. Find a quiet place, sit alone, and think back to the interview you have just had. Were you met as a person by a person? If you met a professional mask who did not let you meet the person behind it, forget it. If you were not met as a unique individual but felt that the same responses you received would have been given to anyone else who happened to make an appointment at that hour, forget it. Did the therapist show concern for your dreams of yourself and seem oriented toward helping you achieve them, or did he seem to feel that he had the correct answers for your life and a blueprint for what you should become? Unless he was oriented to helping you explore *your* dreams and achieve them, forget it. These are the main questions. Unless you get the right answers as you review the session, call up and cancel any appointments you may have made.

The health specialist must be a person who increases the *wellness*, the "spirit-titre," to use psychologist Sidney Jourard's term, of those with whom he comes in contact. This is a matter of personality more than of training, although growth and development can change a person who typically relates to others by making them feel less than they are, into a person who has a positive effect on others. People who diminish others with whom they come in contact do exist. The Yiddish "kvetch" is in this category, as is the character portrayed in the *L'il Abner* comic strip as Joe Btfsplk, who was followed by a constant black cloud. Where he walked plants withered, cows dried up, bridges collapsed, lovers fought, and the healthy became ill. Although the powers of this character were doubtless exaggerated, we have all observed people who "drained" those around them and made everyone in their vicinity feel less instead of more alive. (In my own experience, I can think of a number of neurologists, cardiologists, and nutritionists in particular who had this effect. But this is probably just a personal view. I suspect that the Joe Btfsplks of this world are scattered pretty equally throughout all professions.)

Clearly, when one is seeking a health specialist, those with this type of personality should be avoided. Once one becomes aware that there are those who, in their relationships, increase wellness and others who do the opposite, one can quickly and accurately determine into which group an individual health specialist falls.

From the time health specialists develop mutually respectful working relationships with sickness specialists, the demedicalization of Western society will be under way. We will learn, to use a Biblical analogy, to "render unto Caesar that which belongs to Caesar, and to God that which belongs to God." (Or as the mathematician Norbert Wiener has put it: "unto computers that which belongs to computers and unto man that which belongs to man.") The sickness specialist will help us maintain the *ability* to function; the health specialist will help us determine the *reason*. One will have the role of mechanic to help us fix what is wrong, the other the role of gardener to help us fulfill our potential, for the iris to become the best iris possible, and the willow the best willow. Concerned with our physical, mental, social, and spiritual aspects, holistic medicine will say to us in the haiku of Nikos Kazantzakis:

> I said to the almond tree
> "Sister, speak to me of God."
> And the almond tree blossomed.

WORKING FOR YOUR OWN HEALTH: HOW TO BE YOUR OWN HEALTH SPECIALIST

The concept that the individual damages his health | **6**
when he ignores, represses, or denies expression to
certain parts of his being, or that he allows certain aspects of himself outlet and denies expressing others
at his peril, is far from new. Alcmaeon, the first Greek
to write a medical treatise, to practice dissection, and
to discover that the brain is the central organ of the
sensorimotor system, developed what may be regarded as the first definition of holistic health: "The equal
and cooperative mingling of the separate elements in
human nature ... is health." Alcmaeon's insight is
valid today, although we would use a different classification for the basic elements of human nature. We
would also stress that a different and unique "mingling" is essential for each person's health.

At the center of the modern concept of holistic
medicine is the idea that no one "level," no one domain, of a human being is more "real" than any other. Our nutritional needs are as real and important in
the search for health as are our chemical, medical, interpersonal, creative, and spiritual needs. Each is as
important as the others. If we assume—in the search
for the cure of disease or in the search for health—
that only one level needs to be taken into account,
we will be severely hampered in our efforts.

Even if present surgical techniques were perfect-
ed, the value of a new or repaired heart in the
body of a patient whose life-style remained otherwise unchanged would not be very high.

The general health of populations, then, is not directly dependent on medical services [as they are now de-
fined]. Medical care did not get us out of our own past
troubles and it will not get us out of our present ones.

As we have seen, the theory of "one bacterium, one disease" was always false. Too many people have the germ but
not the disease. But dealing with infectious and communicable diseases, it is a tremendously fruitful idea. It has enabled us to wipe out some of the great killers of human
history and has prevented untold suffering and death. The
problem is that we have expected—and still expect—to use
the same idea in areas where it is not fruitful: in the realm of
degenerative diseases such as heart disease and cancer. Here
the basic fallacy of the concept becomes clear. It simply
does not work.

The British oncologist Sir David Smithers wrote:

Cancer is no more a disease of cells than a traffic jam is a
disease of cars. A lifetime study of the internal combus-
tion engine would not help anyone to understand our
traffic problems. A traffic jam is due to a failure in normal relationships between driven cars and their environment.

What we are beginning to realize is that cells or organs
do not get cancer. People get cancer. If we wish to cure the
disease, we must treat people, not cells or organs.

"If microbes are ever present, yet do not cause disease
until stress, what is the cause of the disease—the microbe
or the stress?" In asking that question, Hans Selye is attempting to point out that this type of "either-or" thinking is long
outdated.

The first artificial-kidney machine failed on the first sixteen patients on which it was tried. It was successful on the
seventeenth, who had decided to change her entire life.

"The first understandable words she spoke . . . were that she was going to divorce her husband, which indeed in time she did. Further recovery was uneventful." Despite countless anecdotes of this type, we still do not take into account in serious procedures (such as surgery, dialysis, and the like) an evaluation of the entire person, and that person's experience in life. A typical research project in this area reports: "The majority of doctors . . . fail to see their patient as a person. . . . [In one study] when asked if they wanted to know more about their patients as individuals, 98 percent of the doctors said no."

It is not only mainline medicine that has concentrated on one level of the total person and ignored the others. Many practitioners of so-called holistic medicine are just as narrow. There is no such thing as a holistic technique or modality. There is only a holistic *attitude*. The most far-out technique can be used, and frequently is, in ways completely opposed to this attitude. For example, an acupuncturist, a homeopath, or a nutritionist who believes that he has *the* answer and that all that anyone needs is his approach is certainly not holistic.

There are, of course, the endless "get-in-shapers." You can see them at gyms and health clubs or, in a slightly different version, at meditation centers, nutrition centers, and health-food stores, and places like Esalen Institute. Endlessly they work at getting one domain of being into shape, at expanding one aspect of themselves. If you ask them what they are getting in shape *for*—how they plan to use the work in one domain to increase the artistic pattern and expression of their whole lives—they look at you blankly. The means has replaced the end. Like the miser who accumulates more and more money and forgets that originally there was a purpose for the money—that he planned to use it for something—they go right on exercising, dieting, or meditating, with no idea of the context of their actions.

I once knew a man who had spent a period of five years

meditating six hours a day, six days a week. Since he had not woven what he had learned into the total context of his life, his meditation had very little effect on him. It probably had about the same effect as if he had spent the time lifting weights in a gymnasium, jogging along a beach, or having his feet massaged. He was the same person at the end of the five years he had been at the beginning, except that now, of course, he could sit in a lotus position for two three-hour periods in a row. It seems like a pretty small gain for the time spent.

This group of "get-in-shapers" is balanced, on the other extreme, by the "holistic athletes" who go from one modality to the next, each time with vast and uncritical enthusiasm, each time certain that this time they are dealing with the level that will change their entire lives and bring them health and happiness. Five years ago they were "into Zen," they sat and meditated (or at least talked about sitting and meditating) for hours on end. They were convinced that this would bring them "enlightenment," which they tended to define in amazingly concrete terms, as if it were a new wardrobe. They felt that it would change everything about themselves. When it failed to do this, they had themselves "Rolfed," massaged, or had a chiropractor adjust their spine. For a time they told everyone how this or that had changed their lives and then presently stopped talking about these treatments when it became plain to themselves and their friends that their lives hadn't changed. Next they went to weekend est sessions where they were harangued, told they were fools and worse for being there, and experienced very full bladders. For a time we all heard how wonderful this had been and how everything in their lives had changed. Then when this made no difference, they took up nutrition and ate only bran and tofu and remarked to all who would listen that since, in terms of defecation, they were no longer "sinkers" but were now "floaters," everything was different. They are now jogging and feel, they will tell you at the drop of an arch, that it changed everything in their lives. In each of these periods, they clearly believed that one level of their being was the real one and all others were of only secondary importance.

Unfortunately we all know people like this, although cure-alls vary from megavitamins to aura balancing and Sufi dancing. None of these people has a "holistic" approach to his own health no matter how often he uses the word. Both holistic athletes and get-in-shapers believe that one level of their being is the "real" and "central" one and that all the others are simply pale reflections of it: that you simply have to be concerned about this one level and everything else will fall into place. In this their bigotry is exactly the same as that of many of the mainline physicians toward whom they express such contempt.

It is not possible within the scope of this book to include a detailed description of each of the adjunctive modalities in use today. And in any case, I am more interested in presenting a way of looking at them and evaluating their relevance for individual needs and health programs. An excellent book that does list and describe many holistic techniques (albeit rather overenthusiastically) is *A Visual Encyclopedia of Unconventional Medicine*. Section headings include: "Comprehensive Systems" (like homeopathy), "Diagnostic Methods" (like biorhythms), "Physical Therapies" (like acupuncture and chiropractic), "Hydrotherapies" (like hot baths and colonic irrigation), "Plant Based Therapies" (like herbal medicine), "Nutrition" (like macrobiotics and high-protein diets), "Mind and Spirit Therapies" (like meditation, psychosynthesis, and gestalt therapy), and "Self-Exercise Therapies" (like yoga and the Alexander technique). Over one hundred different specific techniques are described.

Although it is true that some of the specific techniques are the sheerest kookiness and magical thinking (such as "pyramid energy," or "copper contact") and may be dismissed without further investigation, many of them are serious and complex methodologies that can enable the human organism to use more of its resources to combat disease and grow toward health. There is a vast difference between, for example, such nonsense as iris diagnosis on the one hand, and carefully developed and time-tested methods such as osteopathy, chiropractic, meditation, Zen training, Rolfing, or some nutrition programs on the other.

The references at the end of this chapter will provide a source for material on most of the adjunctive modalities. Although the practitioners of each (who tend to be the best writers on the subject) are likely to be somewhat overenthusiastic about their particular approach, these are reliable sources.

It is possible to formulate some general guidelines that will enable you to evaluate specific modalities and their practitioners, and will be of aid in designing your own program.

1. There is no one program for everyone—such a concept is basically opposed to a cardinal principle of holistic medicine, that the uniqueness in each person is central and important, and that each person should be treated as an individual. Any practitioner who uses the same program design for all—or for a majority—of his or her clients is certainly not practicing holistic medicine.

2. Each modality is designed to help with specific types of problems; it will, if used intelligently, help you with this type of growth. It will not solve *all* your problems. There is no one modality that will do everything you need. That is magic, not the search for health. It seems silly to belabor this obvious point, but it has to be done because so many of those involved in the field do not understand it. They expect that one type of procedure will change everything that needs changing, stimulating, or growing. Since in their overenthusiasm they constantly imply this, it is necessary that in listening to them, or in reading their material, you

bear in mind the limitations of any one form of therapy. Do not expect that your relationship problems will be solved by nutrition, or your creativity-outlet problems by acupuncture. It is true that nutrition or acupuncture may put you in better shape to deal with these other problems, but you still have to deal with them. Jogging may increase your cardiovascular fitness and may tone up your entire body and give you a greater feeling of competence and strength. What you then use these changes for is up to you.

Illustrative of the belief that there is one fundamental domain of experience (level of being) and that all others flow from that is a recent article in the *Health and Diet Times* (March–April, 1981). In discussing cancer, the author of this article came to the conclusion that the only important level to be considered is the nutritional one. The author stated the opinion that the emotional problems so frequently seen before the diagnosis of cancer are due to malnourishment. He concluded that stress is a separate disease syndrome also caused by malnourishment. The article's clear implication was that diet is both the primary cause of cancer and, therefore, its cure: only this aspect of the human being is relevant to the complex disease that is cancer. This is a fairly typical example of how a "holistic" modality can be used in ways opposed to the basic tenets of holistic medicine.

3. There is no free lunch. Every approach that is really effective will take work, organization, planning, consistency. Whether you are involved in a nutrition program, meditating, a movement procedure, or psychotherapy, you are going to have to work at it and stay with it. This is not a puritan attitude that anything worthwhile tastes bad or is uncomfortable. It is rather the knowledge we have gained through long experience that changing one's life is not easy. It would be pleasant to be able to point out a royal road to serenity, strength, health, youthfulness, joy, and zest (and whatever else one thinks desirable). Such a simplistic ap-

proach, no doubt, would help this book sell many more copies. Titles like *How to Achieve Health Through Three Minutes of Easy Relaxation a Day* always do much better than books that say that worthwhile change in your own life must come through long, hard work. Nevertheless if there is one thing that we have learned from thousands of years of experience with the esoteric schools, from the last hundred years of experience with psychotherapy, and from all our experience of holistic medicine, it is that there are very few miracle cures. In fact, you can be sure, in evaluating holistic health practitioners, that if they promise an easy miracle, they are charlatans. If, for example, they promise to change your life in one (or even two) weekends, run, do not walk, to the nearest exit. You are among thieves or fools.

4. Practitioners must not think that they have *the answer*, but must see their own treatment as part of a total approach that includes other levels of your being. They must not only be willing to work with other practitioners who focus on these other levels, but must insist on this. If you are ill and they do not insist that there be also mainline medical coverage of your program, they are dangerous hucksters. Practitioners must meet you as an individual, not as a type of person or a disease. The program must be hand-tailored to your specific personality and situation, not to a general classification into which you are fitted. Practitioners must have a realistic attitude and not insist on a regimen that cannot or will not be carried out. You must be included in the program as an intelligent participant, not as a passive subject.

There has been, in recent years, in the medical and medical ancillary professions, a change from a service orientation to a business orientation. Hence another criterion for choosing a professional, be he a physician or a practitioner of an adjunctive modality: is the physician or practitioner service or business oriented? There are two determining questions in particular you can ask. First, is there a sliding scale of costs? Does he charge less if the client's resources are low? A service-oriented professional does, and the difference in fees is a meaningful one. The second question is even more important. Does he or she give some free time to a clinic or see a certain percentage of clients at no cost? Unless the answer to one of these last is yes, the professional is business oriented.

You may think that while this may be an important consideration in choosing practitioners of adjunctive modalities, you can do just as well—or even, perhaps, better—with a business-oriented physician or surgeon, if he or she is competent. In the long run, this approach is an error. You are not likely to be seen as a unique individual with a unique pancreas, ovary, kidney, or prostate, or whatever the business-oriented specialist is working on. You will be treated more or less as a statistic. In surgery, follow-up will be minimal. (For example, having done the cutting and sewing, the business-oriented surgeon feels that his job is done and he is finished with you. If you are still hurting, that's your problem.) Overall you will probably pay more and get less from a business-oriented professional than from a service-oriented one. Frequently the business oriented specialists claim that the advantage in working with them is in their superior technology and technical skill. First of all, this is rubbish. The best physicians and surgeons (to name only two categories) I know are service oriented. (Sir William Osler wrote: "The practice of medicine is an art, not a trade, a calling, not a business.") Second, the claim would be fine and valid if you were a car that needed fixing, not a person that needs healing. If you prefer being treated like a car, choose your professional accordingly.

In evaluating modes of treatment, it is important to understand that whether a practitioner of an adjunctive modality is considered "paramedical" or "quack" is determined by his relationship to organized medicine and his subservience to the physician, not by what he actually does. The pharmacist is considered to be paramedical, as he makes up his prescriptions under the physician's orders. The nurse and physiotherapist are similarly working under the physician's supervision. The herbalist, the nutritionist, the masseur—and in some cases the midwife—are considered to be quacks because they are not part of this hierarchical system. The masseur may be doing the same things as the physiotherapist, but that is not the point. The difference between being a quack and a paramedical member of the team is not in what you know or do, not in the technology you employ, or in your therapeutic success rate; it is strictly in sociological organization. As I have indicated earlier, the serious adjunctive therapist will insist on working with a physician if there is a disease present. Sometimes, however, this cooperation may be under pretty trying conditions for the adjunctive therapist.

It seems advisable to discuss holistic health programs from two viewpoints: from that of the person who is ill and from that of the person not suffering from a disease. As will be plain from this book, the separation is made for purposes of clarity; in actuality the two types of program have a great deal in common.

1. Holistic programs for the ill person.

If you are ill—and the illness is more than the usual household remedies such as aspirin, bed rest, hot tea, and chicken soup can handle—the first thing you need is a physician's evaluation. Mainline medical treatment comes first, and anyone who skips this step and goes directly to self-treatment has a fool for a patient. Only the physician is equipped to evaluate the potential seriousness of an illness, possible complications, and so forth. Home-reference medical books are not a substitute for a physician's training. Physicians make mistakes and sometimes miss an important diagnosis, but they do this much less frequently than do nonphysicians.

After the diagnosis has been made, however, and after a mainline medical program has been set up, the next step is probably going to be up to you. Physicians, with rare exceptions, usually stop here. If you want to expand the treatment into a holistic approach you will probably have to do it yourself.

As we have said, the first step is to realize that the medical treatment is the place you start, not the place you finish. You start here partly to make as certain as possible that the disease is cured or controlled and does not become worse while you deal with the conditions that made you vulnerable to it. A disease, from the viewpoint of holistic medicine, is a sign that something is wrong with your life. Your task is to find out what that is and to take appropriate action.

There is a tradition in the West that can be very useful in beginning a holistic program. This is to consider the human organism under three categories: body, mind, and spirit. It is true that these are artificial separations, but we need some kind of division of experience in order to begin a search for health, and this is a useful one. ("Only God does not need categories," wrote De Tocqueville. Even Lao-Tsu, writing of the Tao, the basic One of the universe, found it necessary for human purposes to divide it into the *ti-tao*, the Tao of earth, the *jen-tao*, the Tao of man, and the *tien-tao*, the Tao of heaven.)

There are, of course, other ways of categorizing your being than by body-mind-spirit. If you are uncomfortable with this method, choose one of the others. Any one is fine as long as it includes *all* of you. Another example is the division made by some of the German existentialist philosophers: "Relationships with yourself, relationships with others, relationships with the universe." (The *Umwelt*, the *Mitwelt*, and the *Gegenwelt*.) In the first is included your body, mind, feelings; in the second, relationships with other people; in the third, relationships with the universe as a whole and with the meaning of your life. In all serious sets of categories, your social responsibility, your involvement with the fate of the human race, is included. You may include it under mind, spirit, relationships with others, or relationships with the universe. However, it must be included somewhere. We are only psychologically healthy when we are putting some of our energy and concern in this direction, when we are involved not only in our own lives and the lives of others close to us, but also in our own particular version of the Peace Corps.

Using the classic Western mode, you can proceed to ask yourself questions about your life in relation to each of the three categories. First, consider your body. What is your normal life in relation to nutrition, to exercise, to vitamins? Is your body a part of your concern? If not, why not? If so, are you demonstrating this care and concern in your everyday life? If not, what are the appropriate steps to take? For your particular body, age, physique, health level, etc., what are the best things you can do? Try to ignore fads such as jogging. The question is "What does *your* body need?" not "What is popular at the moment?" Walking or yoga may be far better for your particular needs than jogging.

Second, consider your mind. Are you feeding it what it needs, or is it on a diet of the mental equivalent of junk foods? What about your need to learn new things, to use your mind in your own way and style? Have you allowed your mind to stagnate in a daily routine, without feeding it new and stimulating material?

What about your relationships? Are they the correct unique blend that you—one-of-a-kind person—need? Or have they become dull, routine, and meaningless to you? If so, what is the course of action you need to take to keep the world as full of interest, excitement, and surprise as you need it to be? What about your need to *love*? Is this channel of expression free and flowing or blocked like a riverbed full of dead wood and debris?

Do you have the proper balance of relationships and solitude? Each person needs both and each person needs a different percentage of each. (If you can't be alone without depression or anxiety, you are starving some part of yourself. The writer and poet May Sarton has defined loneliness as poverty of the spirit, solitude as richness of the spirit.)

Third, consider your spiritual needs. This is a hard aspect of existence to describe in contemporary America, as we tend to define these needs in terms of a narrow, silly religiosity which often tends to assert that "my symbol of God is the true one; yours is not." When I write here of spiritual needs, I am referring to the *context* of your life and its meaning, your relation to the universe.

Make no mistake about it, a sense of having a place in the larger scheme of things, as all our history shows, is a real and basic human need. We cannot ignore and starve this need and expect to escape unscathed any more than if we ignore the needs of our body or our mind.

The Sufis, who are a group of mystically oriented Moslems, have a story that illustrates this nicely. A Sufi saw a woodchopper go by bearing on his shoulder a freshly cut tree branch. The Sufi said: "See that branch all full of sap and its leaves all green and fresh. It does not know it has been separated from its source. But it will learn, it will learn."

One of the facts discovered by Maslow and his followers in humanistic psychology is that the healthier an individual is psychologically, the greater access he has to his own wellspring of will and desire, the freer he feels inwardly to be himself, the greater the likelihood that he will have the kind of transcendent experiences that will enable him to *know* that he is a part of the total universe, that all human beings are one, and that he is not only his brother's keeper but also his brother. The healthier the person is psychologically, the more at home he is likely to feel in the cosmos and that it is a good home for human beings. The more at ease we are with our own inner life, the more likely we are—in our attitude toward the universe—to move from the viewpoint of Pascal ("The silence of the infinite spaces frightens me!") to the viewpoint of Giordano Bruno ("Out of this world we cannot fall!").

What I am talking about here is the set of beliefs about the nature of a human being and the universe that gives us a set of goals in life and a definition of what makes life worthwhile or not worthwhile. These beliefs help us to determine what is really worth the time and effort of our lives. Unless our lives are in accord with our deepest ethical and spiritual beliefs, we do not feel joy and meaning in our lives and our bodies' resistance to disease is seriously lowered. The biologist René Dubos wrote: ". . . the most compelling factors of the environment, the most commonly involved in the causation of disease, are the goals that the individual sets for himself, often without regard to biological necessity."

If our lives are in accord with our spiritual needs, if we are connected through our actions with the cosmos, we live robustly and joyously "under the roof of eternity." Not only are our bodies more resistant to disease, but we have greater strength to endure those pains and disasters that are a part of being human. "Where there is a 'why,' we can bear any 'how,' " wrote the philosopher Nietzsche.

Knowing the "why" is hard in our twentieth century, a time of transition and change, when the old values and beliefs are dying and the new ones are just being born. Abraham Maslow has written of this dilemma:

> Every age but ours has had its model, its ideal. All of these have been given up by our culture: the saint, the hero, the gentleman, the knight, the mystic. About all we have left is the well-adjusted man without problems, a very pale and doubtful substitute. Perhaps we shall

soon be able to use as our guide and model the fully growing and self fulfilling human being, the one in whom all of his potentialities are coming to full development, the one whose inner nature expresses itself freely, rather than being warped, suppressed, or denied.

This model of the self-fulfilling human being is part of the structure of our present concept of holistic medicine. And it is an important and very useful part. For example, in my years of work with cancer patients, I have constantly faced the problem of what the patient could do to mobilize his host resistance against the pathological process. How could he act so as to bring his own healing and self-repair abilities most effectively to the aid of the medical program?

It has seemed to me that there are three kinds of reasons that a person does not wish to die.

1. Because he is afraid of death or of dying.
2. In order to live for others or to fulfill the demands or expectations of others.
3. To live his own life, to sing the unique song of his own personality.

For reasons I do not fully understand, the body will not mobilize its resources for either or both of the first two reasons. Only for the third will the self-healing and self-recuperative abilities of the individual come strongly into play. When individuals with cancer understand this and begin to search for and fight for their own special music in ways of being, relating, working, creating, they tend to begin to respond much more positively to the medical program. Interestingly enough, I have never seen a case where a person found his own unique way in which his song was not socially positive and did not increase and improve the person's human relationships.

I have written here at somewhat greater length about

spiritual needs than about bodily or mental needs because it is the spiritual needs that most often today tend to be forgotten and slighted. In the gaining of great and detailed technical knowledge about the functioning of the body, we have lost an overall view of what it means to be human. In T. S. Eliot's mournful lament: "How much knowledge have we lost in information."

2. Holistic programs for the person who does not have a disease.

A holistic program for the person without a disease should follow much the same course as one for the ill person, except that it does not start with a physician's evaluation and medical program. The first goal—of curing the disease and trying to prevent its reappearance—is obviously not present. The second goal, of getting the best you can out of your life, of living as fully, as joyfully, as individually as possible, can be shared by both programs.

In his autobiography, *Report to Greco*, Nikos Kazantzakis wrote: "We must leave the earth not like scourged, tearful slaves, but like kings who rise from the table with no further wants, after having eaten and drunk to the full."

As in the program for the person with a disease, we would ask ourselves questions about the different realms of our existence: the physical, the mental, the spiritual. In each realm we would explore and try to determine in which realm we needed to make changes.

In doing this, it is important to be aware that we are not static, fixed beings, but are continually developing. What is right and fulfilling for us in one period of our lives is not necessarily so in another. Our existence is a living room, not a waiting room. We are not the same as we were previously, nor will we be in the future what we are now, and our needs are not the same. A diet of mother's milk, as a rather extreme example, is perfect for a baby. A few years later such a diet would be lacking in some essential ingredients and would rapidly lead to one of the deficiency diseases.

We must, in this search, look at ourselves with fresh and open eyes and without fixed preconceptions. Freud once wrote: "The essence of analysis is surprise." This is true of all human growth, with or without the aid of psychotherapy. If we do not allow ourselves to be surprised as we evaluate ourselves, we will see and learn nothing new. Long ago, Heraclitus warned us, "Unless we expect the unexpected, we will never find it." Human life—and the psychologically healthier a person is, the more this is true—is as full of the unexpected and surprising as is the first sunrise seen through the eyes of a child.

There is no safety and happiness within walls for human beings. We must grow or stagnate. Life is risking, changing, becoming. Happiness for us does not consist in the safety of a clam, but in using ourselves as completely as possible in our own way. It consists in the act of creating ourselves. We may, of course, think that we are creating something else— a family, a cathedral, a space shuttle, a business, or a law practice. If we are involved not only in the thing itself, but also in our own creation of self, we are probably happy, although far too busy to think about it.

One of the most important aspects of a holistic health approach is to learn to listen to signals from our own organism and to treat them as important information. Whether one is in psychotherapy and learning to listen to the faint music of one's own song to sing, whether these messages come in the form of intuitions, preferences, or dreams, or whether one is in a sensory-awareness session learning to listen to one's own muscles, the same rule applies: This is important information and to be reacted to as such. If you are in a nutrition center where all they eat is rice and carbohydrates and you keep longing for a particular food—say, fried chicken—your body is telling you something. We ignore such messages at our peril. Take an occasional one-meal vacation from the diet and have some fried chicken. You may accomplish your goals at the nutrition center a little more slowly, but you are more likely to stay on the diet to reach them and you are also likely to save yourself a lot of future trouble by learning to respond to valid bodily signals.

If you have a cancer and are in the midst of a chemotherapy program, you may experience overwhelming feelings that the chemicals used are damaging your body. These are different feelings from those indicating that the drugs are terribly unpleasant, that they constantly make you nauseated, or that you are fed up with them. It is a clear set of feelings—and you will recognize them if you are aware of the possibility of having them—that the chemicals are doing damage to you. If you have these feelings, they should be treated as important. Tell your physician about them and do not accept his reassurance. They are *your* very individual body and your feelings, and you are the only one who can be aware of them. Tell the physician that you want a new program designed using different chemicals. Other programs do exist and so do other physicians. People have died from chemotherapy because they ignored these kinds of signals.

The same rule applies to all of mainline medicine and all the adjunctive modalities. If you are in a psychotherapy program and feel worse after the sessions most of the time, get another therapist. The proof of the pudding is in the eating and the proof of psychotherapy is—at least a majority of the time—in your feeling better and more at home with yourself, others, and the world after a session than you did before. If you are in a meditation program and the meditations make you feel worse, or if you feel that you are hurting yourself by doing them, stop.

Some years ago, I enrolled in a developmental program called the Gurdjieff "Work." The program includes a fairly heavy meditation schedule. There is one particular kind of meditation central to the program—a form of meditation where you keep your mind highly aware of yourself and everything you are doing. It is called "self-remembering." I understood the rationale of this form of meditation, why it was constructed in the way it was, and why it was included in the program, and I found that this was a meditation that I was able to do exceptionally well. Each time I finished, however, I had two conflicting feelings. The first was that of being in a "charged up," "put together" state. The second was that I had ingested some sort of poison that would damage me. I went to the head of the program for an explanation and an alternative approach that would not give me the second feeling. When he had neither to offer, but said just to trust him and continue to follow his instructions, I left the program and sought ways of personal growth in other developmental systems. Eventually I found a good program for myself based on some of the Western meditational systems. Like most of the people who leave hospitals against medical advice, I have never regretted it.

If you are in a nutrition center where all they serve is brown rice and beans and you have the clear feeling that this is bad for your body, leave the center. Remember, you are a unique individual and your body reacts in a unique way. Since the practitioners of the adjunctive modalities frequently ignore this point, you will have to be the one who stays keenly aware of it. Practitioners and physicians alike tend to become so involved in the particular approach they are using that they forget the individuality of each person. Until we train health specialists, you will have to be on your own.

One last general comment about holistic health programs: They must be reasonable. By this I mean that a program must be one you will do, not just one you wish you would do. I would, for example, like to be a person who meditates an hour a day. I am not. If I set up a program calling for an hour of meditation a day, I will not follow it. I will skip it one day and skimp on it the next. Presently I will give it up entirely. I am a person who *will* follow a program of twenty minutes of meditation six times a week. That program, for me, is *reasonable*, in terms of who I am at this point in my own development.

Recently a cancer patient of mine went to a "holistic health center" where they specialized in nutrition. This woman was quite wealthy, and had a full-time private nurse. She took the tests, including a full chemical analysis of her hair, at the center, and they devised a nutritional and general gastrointestinal program for her. It included a great many special foods, blended concoctions, coffee enemas, raw liver juice, and vitamins. After I had examined the large sheets of paper describing what she should prepare, eat, or do during each twenty-four-hour period, the patient asked me what I thought of the program. I replied that even without analyzing the nutritional and biochemical aspects of the program, I could say it was useless. She simply was not going to follow it. The patient replied that she and the nurse had gone over it in detail and come to the conclusion that if the nurse arrived a half hour earlier each day and the two of them then spent the entire day on it, they could just barely keep up with the schedule. The program might have been "reasonable" for a clinic or hospital inpatient with access to a kitchen staff, but it was completely unreasonable for outpatients.

It is important to set up a program that you actually will do. A less ambitious program you will follow is vastly more effective than a more complex program you won't.

The adjunctive therapist must focus on two separate aspects of the problem when dealing with a particular patient. The first is: "What does this patient *need*?" The second is: "Who is this patient and what will he *do*?" Both must be understood if the program is to be realistic.

Recently I observed a highly competent nutritionist working with a woman with a fairly severe heart condition. The nutritionist worked out a dietary program admirably suited to the disease. There was, it turned out, only one problem. It was not suited to the patient. For example, the program included a procedure each morning in which the patient would have to blend together various raw vegetables and drink the result while it was still fresh. This particular patient went to work early each morning and awoke with her mind on the problems of the day. She could make a cup of coffee and drink it with food prepared the night before, but found it difficult to focus on preparing elaborate food that early in the day. It was so difficult for her to do this that she simply was not going to continue this program.

If the nutritionist had spent as much time on the question of who this patient was and what she would do, as she spent on the problem of her nutritional needs, a program could have been worked out that would be the best possible compromise. It would have been a sensible program, and consequently the patient would not have abandoned the nutritional approach. As one example, the blended vegetables could have been made and drunk at supper.

The nutritionist saw the importance of the nutritional domain, but forgot the rest of the patient. A holistic modality was being used in a nonholistic manner.

The same problem is seen in many of the esoteric meditative schools such as Zen Buddhism, Sufism, and so on. A person might come to an intensive training group and work hard and for long hours at meditation. Under group auspices and for a limited period, the work seems reasonable. The person then might be given a meditation program to do at home. Since programs are not designed for each individual and one general program is given for all, a large percentage of the students find, after they have returned home, that it is not a program they will follow. They drop the whole approach.

Part of the reason for this narrowness on the part of

many adjunctive therapists is the fact that when we work at something and pour our efforts into it, our estimation of its importance tends to increase. We tend to become so involved that we see the patient only through the lens of our particular interest. We tend more and more to believe that we have found *the* answer and that if the patient uses our approach correctly, everything will be fine. This is as true of surgeons (who have a nasty tendency to believe that if a particular operation does not achieve the desired results, then a follow-up operation that removes more tissue or the next organ *will* work) as it is of megavitamin enthusiasts, who believe that if 1,000 units of vitamin C are good, 2,000 are twice as good. Most of us see *our* approach as correct and other approaches as much less important or efficacious.

When it was pointed out to the nutritionist in the previous example that she was not taking the other levels of the patient's existence into account, she replied, "But, Dr. LeShan, you do not know how effective nutrition is." (You could easily substitute "psychotherapy," "chiropractic," "meditation," "yoga," or any other adjunctive modality for "nutrition.") These practitioners are not trying to bring about the basic change that a holistic viewpoint would imply. They simply believe that *their* approach should replace mainline medicine as the orthodox healing art and that mainline medicine should then assume a secondary role. They no more see the patient as functioning on a number of equally important levels than does the orthodox physician.

Although it is important that the practitioner of an adjunctive modality be realistic and shape a program that the client will follow, it is also important that the client be realistic and evaluate his or her own limits. Generally we are willing to face and accept far more discomfort and change in our daily lives from mainline medicine than we are willing to accept from the adjunctive modalities. The client must decide if the refusal to follow an adjunctive program is due to a realistic self-appraisal or to a neurotic and petulant resistance to changing. Is he reacting to a program that is not destined for him as a specific individual, or is he insisting that he attain his goals with no difficulty or discomfort?

I have discussed both those who are using holistic medicine for a specific illness and those who are illness free. But there are two other relevant classes of people, and I wish to address them here.

First, there are those who feel ill, but are unable to get a diagnosis. The physician responds with a shrug or the general attitude of "I can't find anything wrong, let's wait." (Basically the physician seems to be saying, "You're not sick enough. Come back when things progress further.") The patient knows that something is the matter, but whatever it is does not show up on physical examinations or tests. The physician may suggest a tranquilizer or a vacation, or some other vague remedy that does not seem to have anything to do with the problem.

The first thing to do, of course, is to check with a second (and possibly a third) physician. You may have consulted a turkey the first time. If second and third physicians are unable to arrive at a specific diagnosis, even though you know that you feel ill, then you will have to take the situation into your own hands. It is time to do some general upgrading of your life. Nutritional programs, exercise programs, and the type of self-examination I have described as desirable for the first two classes of people dealt with in this section, are now indicated.

If you don't wait for the condition to develop further, but undertake this general upgrading, the condition may go away. You may never find out what it was, but is that so important? If the condition does develop, you will be in far better shape to deal with it. The better shape your entire organism is in, the better you can cope with disease and the less likely disease is to appear at all.

There is another group of individuals for whom a diagnosis has been made, but for whom mainline medicine can do little. It is wise for these individuals to examine the adjunctive modalities immediately and see if they have anything to offer. Very often the long experience of adjunctive therapists has shown them that their methods are applicable to certain conditions that the mainline physician cannot treat. It is now obvious (although just a few years ago it was not) that if you are subject to migraines you do not have either to bear them or else go around heavily drugged, which is about all that orthodox medical training indicates. You can go to a psychotherapist, for example. Biofeedback procedures and relaxation techniques have often been very useful. The same is true of lower-back pain. Formerly, major surgery that was often useless was the only alternative to chronic discomfort. In many cases, this condition responds to psychotherapy, chiropractic, movement therapy, or meditation.

A physician's diagnosis of obesity does not mean that this is a condition physicians are equipped to deal with. Nutritionists and psychotherapists (and frequently volleyball coaches) often are far more effective in dealing with this problem.

Osteoporosis, a condition in which the calcium is leached out of the bones, leaving them weak and breakable, is a diagnosis not treatable successfully by mainline medicine. It does, however, sometimes respond to a combination of carefully monitored nutrition and exercise programs. If I had multiple sclerosis, another condition not treatable by mainline medicine, I would certainly explore a nutrition approach and a variety of other adjunctive methods.

While orthodox medicine is *essential* for diagnosis, it may or may not be useful for treatment. After diagnosis of such conditions as the ones cited above, another modality would be the mainline approach and orthodox medicine the adjunctive modality.

It is time now to discuss a number of cases of the actual practice of holistic medicine. These will be presented in the following chapter.

THE PRACTICE OF HOLISTIC MEDICINE: CASE HISTORIES AND DEMONSTRATIONS OF THE METHOD

> Of all the wonders, none is more wonderful than man. . . . He has learned the art of speech and wind-swift thought and living in neighborliness. And how to build shelter against cold, refuge from rain. He can always help himself: he faces no future helpless. There is only death he cannot ultimately escape. He has contrived refuge from illness once beyond all cure.
>
> SOPHOCLES—*Antigone*

7

In the previous chapters, I have discussed the modern field of holistic medicine in general terms. It is now time to put some flesh on these rather sparse bones and to discuss how holistic medicine can work in actual practice: how to work with a health specialist if one is available, or how to function as your own health specialist. In this chapter, I will illustrate what holistic health and medicine is all about with a number of case histories of individuals who have used holistic approaches. All four of the classes described previously will be covered: those who have a specific disease that is treatable by mainline medicine; those who are illness free; those who are ill and have symptoms, but for whom no diagnosis can be found; and those who have a disease not treatable by mainline medicine. In the following chapter, I will discuss the problem of functioning successfully when you are in a hospital. These two chapters should make concrete what I have so far written about in theoretical terms.

In the case histories there will be mention of various adjunctive therapies used by the person described. I have included a short (and woefully inadequate) description of each of the modalities mentioned. This will serve as an introduction to the types that are available today. In effect, it is a sort of sampler of them. For further details, both of these methods and of the many others that are presently available, I would recommend the books listed in the notes for chapter 6 at the end of this book.

Let us look now at how a number of individuals have used modern holistic medicine in their search for health. The first case is that of a woman with a mild, but painful, condition which could be treated and relieved, but not cured, by mainline medicine:

R. was a divorced woman in her late forties. She worked for an industrial company as office manager and head of the typing pool. She "rather enjoyed" her work and had no desire to change it. Her personal relationships consisted of several close women, each of whom she saw for lunch or dinner and theater every few weeks, a number of affairs of from six months to a year's duration, and an intermittent sexual relationship with her ex-husband. (About 30 percent of divorced couples continue to sleep together occasionally.) Her major physical exercise consisted of walking to and from work (a distance of about a mile) whenever New York weather permitted.

On the average of twice a year she would have lower-back pain of an intensity that would make it necessary for her to remain in bed for two to three weeks. These attacks would come on suddenly with no apparent cause and would be agonizing. The pain was reduced by a combination of Valium and Darvon, the use of wet heating pads, and as little movement as possible. Although several specialists she had consulted had suggested surgery, her general practitioner was against the idea, saying that in his experience it was ineffective for conditions like hers, and sometimes even made matters worse. Since she disliked the idea of surgery, she followed his advice.

Five years ago, she heard of a holistic health center that had opened in her neighborhood, and after a particularly bad attack of back pain, she phoned them and made an appointment.

After a medical report had been forwarded to them by her GP (some holistic health centers follow this procedure, some do their own physical workups, and some rely on both) she had a long discussion with their chief counselor. She decided to examine the various spheres of her life and see which were not fully nourished. This was done in a series of sessions with a health specialist at the center.

As a result of this examination, she made a number of decisions. She started "shopping" for a psychotherapist to explore her inner world, her "inscape," in John Donne's phrase, with which she met the "landscape" of the outer world. She did not find the two psychotherapists at the center particularly sympathetic and, after one session with each, decided to look further. As soon as she started to talk with the fourth therapist she consulted, an older, European-trained woman psychiatrist, who had a viewpoint strongly influenced by the teachings of Viktor Frankl, she had an immediate sense of recognition and of "coming home." They worked together twice a week for nearly two years.

Becoming aware that she needed work on the level of the body, she also started once-a-week sessions with a teacher of the Alexander technique. This is a gentle method for becoming aware of the ways our positions (as in sitting, standing, and walking) express and reinforce our tensions and habits, and vary from the ways that are least stressful and most natural for us. In the words of one of its leading practitioners—Ilana Rubenfeld—it is "learning to use rather than misuse the body." Students learn how their "body/mind 'speaks' and how to 'listen' to ourselves and others in a flowing and congruent manner."

In his Nobel Prize acceptance speech in 1973, Nikolaas Tinbergen described the effect that the Alexander technique had had on himself, his wife, and his daughter. They noted ". . . very striking improvements in blood pressure, breathing, depth of sleep, overall cheerfulness and mental alertness, resilience against outside pressure, and also in refined skill such as playing a musical instrument. . . . Although no one would claim . . . [it] is a cure-all in every case, there is no doubt that it often does have profound and beneficial effects . . . in both the mental and the emotional sphere."

R. had two discussions with the nutritionist at the center. Following this, she generally upgraded her diet and added a daily vitamin and mineral supplement.

In view of the spiritual deficiencies revealed in the survey of her life, R. also started teaching two evenings a week at the Fortune Society, an organization of ex-convicts who have turned their lives around and are trying to help others to do the same. Their success rate is very high. (The rate of return to prison for people associated with them is .07 percent. The national rate for ex-convicts is 75 percent.) Among their programs is a literacy program for those ex-offenders who are handicapped by never having learned to read and write well enough to function effectively in society. R. works in this program and finds that she enjoys it, looks forward to the evening she will be teaching, and that, in doing this, she is nourishing a previously undernourished part of herself.

She has developed an interest in serious music, has a rather good record collection, and attends a subscription series of concerts each winter. She took flute lessons for about a year, but then began to find the practicing tedious and gave it up.

After the first six months of the new program, her lower-back pain attacks lessened in intensity and frequency and she has had none in the past two and a half years. She reports much more energy and vitality than ever before, and rates her present life as "very satisfactory."

In this case history we see an approach to health in

three different realms—body, mind and emotions, and spirit—and an upgrading in each. In her work with the Fortune
Society, R. was expressing that side of her being that needed context, meaning, and an identification with more than
herself, with a larger view. Spiritual development does not
mean visions and enlightenments. Indeed, most mystics
warn against taking these seriously. It means knowing that
you are a part of the total One of the cosmos and this is
better done through action than ecstasy. The Talmud says,
"Who heals one soul, it is as if he healed the whole world.
Who harms one soul, it is as if he harms the entire world."
It was *this* spiritual path that R. was taking, and it was right
for her.

The end result was a remission of the disease process,
an end of feeling ill, and a greatly heightened participation
in her own life. We see the same pattern of highly individualized action in the next case, a man with a far more serious condition.

T. was a very successful executive in his mid-forties. He
worked for a large company, and had been promised a major promotion within a year. This was the job he had been
aiming for since he had first joined the company seventeen
years before. He had been married for fifteen years to a
chic, bright, and ambitious career woman. He described the
marriage as "okay, no problems," and she concurred with
this opinion. Both loved skiing and they took regular vacations in Switzerland. The center of his world was his work,
at which he was very good indeed. He was liked and admired by subordinates, colleagues, and superiors.

Two months before he was to move into the new job, a
number of sudden symptoms brought him to seek medical
help. A rapidly growing Hodgkin's disease (cancer of the
lymphatic system) was diagnosed. At that time (the early
1960s) the prognosis for this condition was extremely poor,
although now it is almost 85 percent curable. The Hodgkins
Institute in New York City had at that time no cases of five-

year survival in its records. T. was started on a radiation program. (This, with cortisone and nitrogen mustard treatment, was all that mainline medicine had to offer at the time.) During the course of treatment, he was referred to the staff psychologist as part of a research program that was being conducted. After the exploratory interview, he told the psychologist that he felt his cancer "had something to do with, maybe was caused by, my emotions." (Twenty years ago the idea that it is fruitful to look at cancer as a disease of the whole organism, not as a set of problems of a group of cells—in short, that people get cancer and it is people who must be treated—was known to very few physicians, although a great many cancer patients were aware of it.)

The psychologist at the hospital where T. was being treated as an outpatient was experimenting with the health-therapist concept and, in this case, functioned in that role. A psychotherapy program was started. Encouraged to take his destiny into his own hands, he went to a nearby medical library and learned all he could about Hodgkin's disease. Not at all satisfied with what mainline medicine had to offer and the extremely poor prognosis that was predicted for his condition, he decided to look further. He started by consulting an osteopath.

The osteopathic physician places great emphasis on the self-healing abilities of the individual and on the "structure function principle." In most states the O.D. degree is considered to be equal to the M.D. and the osteopath can prescribe and administer drugs and perform surgery when he or she believes them to be indicated. The structure-function principle states that diseased function is usually a result of displaced structure interfering with normal nerve and blood-system functioning. Osteopathy, therefore, stresses musculoskeletal manipulation, which often cures not only the structural problem (such as out-of-line vertebrae) but the corresponding functional or physiological problems as well.

The osteopath brings to disease and health problems

the standard medical armamentarium plus a strong belief in the self-healing abilities of the body, and a specialized manipulation technique that often permits these abilities to function at a higher level.

The osteopath that T. saw recommended that he continue the radiation program prescribed by his oncologist and, in addition, prescribed a number of sessions of osteopathic manipulation. T. reported that the treatments made him feel a great deal better and that he had more energy after the series.

It was hard at the time to find a nutritionist who had common sense, training, and experience with life-threatening diseases, but after some search T. managed to do so. He went on a strict vegetarian diet with heavy vitamin and mineral supplements. The diet was not one that would be recommended by most nutritionists today, but it seemed to be the best advice he could get at the time.

In addition, T. began to work daily with the Simonton technique, an adjunctive method specifically designed to stimulate his self-healing abilities and to bring them to the aid of the mainline medical program. In this specialized meditation method one visualizes both the cancer cells and the self-defense forces in a concrete, "cartoon" fashion, and then concentrates on imagining a conflict between them, with the cancer cells being defeated. Thus one might (if this were the image one arrived at naturally, and which felt comfortable) visualize the healing forces as armored Crusader knights attacking and killing the cancer cells in the form of dragons. Originated by Carl Simonton, M.D. (who found that patients who did this meditation consistently and had radiation responded better than control groups who only received radiation), it has proved widely useful as an adjunctive modality for cancer treatment. Physicians and others who teach this visualization method are now available, as are Simonton's book (*Getting Well Again*) and training cassettes.

During psychotherapy, it rapidly became apparent to T.

that his marriage was an empty shell. Both he and his wife had settled for something very far from ideal. There was little to hold them together besides habit and T.'s belief (which his wife apparently shared) that nothing better was possible. An exploration was made of his deep despair about ever attaining any really loving relationship. At one point he said: "You know how it is, Doc, with a house with no insulation. No matter how much heat you put into it, you can't get warm. You can only do that by having some of the heat reflected back at you. I always knew that that's how it was with me in life. No matter how hard I tried, no matter how much heat I put out, I would never be able to get warm." Working through and dissipating this despair stemming from early childhood experiences was a long and painful task.

When he began to realize how little he had settled for in his marriage, he and his wife began to examine the situation together and—for the first time—to really talk about it. They went to a marriage counselor together and had several sessions with him. At the same time, she was offered a better job if she would move to another city. This seemed to clinch it for both of them and they divorced in an amiable manner. Both seemed to be quite relieved.

For a time after the divorce T. felt that he wanted no relationships other than those in his work. This desire was explored in the psychotherapeutic sessions and the fear behind it was accepted and worked through. He then began to date and saw a number of women a few times each. After about a year, one relationship developed into an affair and then a marriage. The second wife is much more open and loving than the first. Reminded of his earlier remark about insulation, he grinned and said he felt "pretty warm now."

Psychotherapeutic exploration was also done in the work area. T. realized that the job he had been aiming at all those years now seemed to him to be a dead end. He felt that instead of producing the endless challenge and stimulation that he had, all these years, fantasied that it would, the job probably would become boring in a year or two, like all the other jobs he had had. Once he had been through a cycle of the major problems of a job a couple of times, he felt bored and ready to move on. After this new job, there would be no place to move to, and he would be "all dressed up with no place to go. Ever!"

When T. began to understand his feelings about work, he also began to see the fallacy of his presuppositions. The new job was one of which he could make anything he wanted, and his superiors were clearly hoping that he would be continuously creative and would develop in new ways. The despair over work also began to disappear. (The despair over both the job and his emotional relationships, the feeling of being at a dead end in both, and the "sudden" appearance of a very severe disease, reminded the therapist of Jung's statement, "When an inner situation is not made conscious, it appears outside as fate." At one point in a session, he mentioned this and T. thought about it for a very long minute, and nodded in complete and sad agreement.)

The therapist kept pointing out to him that he was doing beautifully in the spheres of his existence directly affected by the psychotherapeutic process, but that there were at least two other spheres he was neglecting—the physical and the spiritual. In the physical realm, the nutritional program was a beginning, but only that. Checking each time with his oncologist, he experimented with a number of forms of physical activity. He joined a well-known New York athletic club in which there were a large number of activities and classes in everything from yoga to judo. He tried a number of these in an attempt to find one that felt right for this period of his life and that would help him with the necessary upgrading of his physical being. After trying several that were not relevant for him, he found that swimming laps in the local pool was exactly what he wanted. He would slowly swim dozens of laps with his mind focused only on the swimming, completely aware of what he was doing, and not allowing himself to be distracted. He would generally emerge from the pool feeling slightly "high," "well put together," and calm and energetic. He found that he wanted to do this four times a week before going to work and that this program was—at this point in his development—right for him.

Understanding (intellectually only at this point) that he was not expressing or nourishing the spiritual part of his nature, and that this was not permissible for him, not something from which he could escape unscathed, he began to try to discover and experience this part of himself. He knew that he was searching for a larger context to his life and that this was expressed in different ways by different people: some in a direct comprehension of their oneness with the cosmos; some in an identification with the human race as a whole and in working in a specific way for its development; and some, ideally, with both. He attended several Catholic retreats and found them "interesting" and "pleasant," but did not feel that they had real meaning for him. Some Zen seminars where the participants sat most of the day—in what for him, at least, was an uncomfortable position—he found interesting, but not pleasant. After a number of experiments, he decided that an Eastern breath-counting meditation was what he was looking for and started doing this regularly one half hour each day. He found that when he did this he felt better and more energetic all day, less "flappable," and more at home with himself and others.

This meditation is done by getting into a comfortable position and simply counting one's exhalations to "four" and then starting over again. Every attempt is made to remain as alert and awake, as completely conscious of what one is doing, as possible. As soon as the mind drifts off and becomes aware of something else, it is brought back to the task as firmly and as gently as possible. One treats oneself as one would wish to be able to treat a beloved child, demanding the best, but with love, compassion, and humor. The task is not to learn how to meditate well (*no one* ever does that) but to learn to catch oneself more and more quickly when the mind drifts off the task, and bring it back more rapidly, firmly, and lovingly. As with the other disciplined meditations, this work trains and tunes the mind as working in a gymnasium disciplines and tunes the body. If performed conscientiously and over a long period of time, it will also lead to transcendental understandings in which one begins to comprehend deeply our oneness with the entire cosmos and to *know* that our alienation and separation are illusions. Working regularly with a disciplined meditation program helps one function more efficiently in this world of the "many" and also in the world of the "One."

About a year after T. started working on the meditation program, he attended a meeting of the American Association for the United Nations to which a colleague had invited him. He found that he responded to their approach and became interested in their work. He is now a senior officer in one of the chapters of this organization and is on several committees on the national level.

The Hodgkin's disease responded well to the radiation program. The tumors regressed and did not reappear for about six months. A number of them then became apparent to X-ray and a further course of radiation was prescribed. The tumors again disappeared and have not, in the seventeen years since then, reappeared.

T. has, in this time, changed both his exercise and his meditation program several times. What is right for us in one period of our development is not necessarily right in another. He has changed his diet several times, both because of new information and because of his own needs. He worked at the job he was promoted to for about eight years and then moved to another company at a higher position. He enjoys his work. His marriage is a good one and he has two children, one of them an adopted Korean boy. He rates his life as "diverse, exciting, and fascinating. The only problem I have is that there are only twenty-four hours in a day and I have about thirty-six hours of things I like to do."

Here again we see a pattern of individualized upgrading of life in as many domains as possible. T. took responsibility for his own life and sought help from as many teachers and therapists as he felt necessary. The holistic approach does not mean using an adjunctive modality instead of mainline medicine when there is a problem. (Although this is often the picture presented by those practitioners of adjunctive modalities who feel themselves to be in a power struggle with mainline medicine. These persons are fighting for control, not trying to establish a new approach to health.)

The holistic approach is rather illustrated in these case histories of individuals who played an active and knowledgeable part in designing unique and individual programs for themselves, programs that dealt with as many levels of their being as possible and were built on the assumption that they had strong self-healing and self-repair abilities that could be mobilized under the proper conditions.

One of the errors of mainline medicine is that "health" is the absence of disease, and that one need therefore only use medical methods—mainline or adjunctive—when actually ill. (Maimonides wrote, "He is a great fool who believes he only needs a physician when he is ill.") The holistic approach to health is that it is far more than the absence of disease, it is a *process* of approaching one's fullest, most zestful, and joyful participation in every aspect of one's own life. The farther along one is on the path to this participation, the more one is using this method.

The following case history is included as an example of someone who, with no disease present, used this approach to life.

M. was in his late thirties and divorced. He had one child, who was now in her early teens, lived with her mother, and saw M. on occasional weekends and holidays. He was an associate professor of business management in a middle-sized college in a large East Coast city.

There was nothing in particular wrong with him physically, but—as he put it later—"There was nothing particularly right with me or my life, either." He spent his vacations at singles' hotels in the mountains, which, as he described them, were "pleasantly promiscuous."

(It must be remembered that terms like "promiscuous" tell us more about the person using them than they do about the activity they are used to describe. They are relative, not absolute, descriptions. In a study of a similar loaded term, a large group of physicians were given a questionnaire about their health, which included a question about their weight. A few weeks later they were given a questionnaire about medical matters that included a question about their definition of *obesity*. Nearly all of them defined an obese person as one who weighed a little more than they did.)

M. had several single women friends and generally mild, rather friendly, long-term affairs with two of them. He would have four to six shorter affairs each year. These varied from a weekend to a month or two in length. He had no close men friends. He was witty and intelligent and was frequently invited to dinner parties by relatives or acquaintances who either needed an extra man for the evening or else had a woman friend or relative they wanted him to meet. He enjoyed these social events, but made sure "that they came to nothing." He had been once to a swingers' club that featured a nightly orgy, but never returned. When questioned about this, he would tell the story of Voltaire, who had been invited to an orgy, accepted, acquitted himself magnificently, and refused to go again with the statement, "Once a philosopher, twice a pervert."

When the fad was at its height, he took up jogging and did this several times a week. Later, in keeping with many in his social class, he switched to tennis.

In short—in the words Tolstoi used to describe the life

of Ivan Ilych—"his life was most ordinary and therefore most terrible." It was pleasant, highly socially acceptable, busy, and essentially meaningless. He had found a way of life that made no demands on him and that was unrelated to his own particular being.

The summer he was thirty-nine he decided to take part of his vacation on a walking tour of New England instead of in his usual manner. (He recently had seen the original *Goodbye, Mr. Chips* on television, in which Robert Donat, leading a dull life as a teacher in an English preparatory school, meets Greer Garson on a walking tour of the Alps and this event changes his entire life. M. later felt that this had influenced his decision.) Walking alone for three weeks, he began to feel that his life was somehow empty, that something was missing. Walking all day in the crisp spring air of Vermont and New Hampshire, he felt at once exhilarated and depressed. He knew that he needed something new, but could form no idea of what it might be.

What he did not realize at this time was that he was going through what the psychiatrist Carl Jung called the "second adolescence." From Jung's viewpoint, those who are lucky enough to go through this generally do so between thirty-five and fifty. During the process, those who are able to succeed in the developmental task of this period find themselves shifting their primary life orientation from concern with the opinions of others to concern with the growth of the self.

On his return to the city, he made an appointment with a psychiatrist he had met at a party a year before. This man had impressed him as "someone who seemed to be really anchored in the world." As they worked together, the realization grew in him that he had adjusted himself to life rather than the other way around. In the process he had completely lost sight of himself as an individual.

He began to explore with the therapist who *he* was. Among the first things that he found out was that he was a person who enjoyed learning new things, but had "forgotten" this and had fed his mind no new nourishment for a long time. Because of his interest in business management, he began to read (and to audit some courses in his own and a nearby university) about the history of that field and its relationships to other aspects of cultural development. In two years, he found, rather to his surprise, that he was teaching several new courses (he had been teaching the same ones over and over for nearly fifteen years), that he had published several papers in his new field of interest, and had something of a reputation as an expert in it.

The exploration of his inner life led him to explore his deep fear of serious relationships and, indeed, of letting himself be deeply committed to anything. His relationship with his daughter improved markedly, as did his relationship with one of the two women with whom he had been having an affair. They are now living together and both see it as a "probably permanent" arrangement.

He has rediscovered a college interest in jazz music of the twenties and thirties, and gets a good deal of enjoyment from it. He tried, at the therapist's suggestion, both Zen and yoga, but found that they did not seem relevant to who he was and where he was in his development. He has experimented with a number of physical approaches from karate to weight lifting and finally found one that he enjoys and that refreshes and invigorates him. This is Tai-chi, an ancient Chinese exercise system designed to integrate all the aspects of the person through a series of flowing movements on which the mind is completely focused. These movements, originally taken from the natural movements of animals and birds, appear to the observer as a dance of continuous postures set to the rhythm of slow, deep breathing. It is a movement meditation designed to use gently every muscle in the body and to stimulate the circulation and the flow of energies in the body. It is both a physical exercise and a meditation. With practice it leads to a "passive exhilaration," a "calm excitement," and a sense of the unity of oneself and the universe.

Over his therapist's desk there was a sampler with the words "If we heal the cosmos, we heal ourselves. If we heal ourselves, we heal the cosmos." He had gradually understood the need for *context* in his life; the need for participation in the human race. He finds a great deal of satisfaction, and the easing of a need he did not earlier know was there, in working two evenings a week as the volunteer business manager of an ecology organization.

He is now so engaged in and committed to his life that he does not ask himself much if he is enjoying it: he *knows* its meaning and value. He says with a laugh, "I wonder what my next walking trip will lead to."

As the case histories illustrate, one of the cardinal principles of the new methodology is the requirement of activity on the part of the person involved. You must be active and seek for yourself. Find out what therapies are available and what are their likely results. It is relevant that the word "cure" derives from the same root as the word "curiosity." Be "curious" and take your destiny into your own hands. It is a lot safer there than in the hands of strangers.

There is a second principle involved that is repeatedly illustrated here: there are no basic contradictions between methods that seek to upgrade various domains of your being. You do not do harm to one domain by doing good to another. As a specific example of this, E. Cheraskin—one of the leading modern experts in holistic health—has pointed out in a number of books and papers that there is no diet that is good for only one disease. A diet is either good for you or it is not. It is not good for your teeth and bad for your hemorrhoids or vice versa. If something is bad for your teeth, it is bad for the rest of you also. In his words: "The point being stressed is that common sense, if nothing else, would indeed suggest that if sugar is bad for the top of your body, it is equally bad for the bottom of your body.

People do not walk around rotting from the waist up and healing from the waist down."

Cheraskin goes on to point out that a diet may be good for you or not good for you, but there is no one diet for everyone. Each person has individual needs. For example, if you live in a city (and therefore inhale a lot of lead) you need more vitamin C, which is a good chelating agent (an agent that unites with the lead and forms a substance that the body can excrete). If you smoke, or take aspirin, or are on the pill, you also need more, as these things interfere with your ability to metabolize vitamin C. If you do all four, you certainly need a lot more vitamin C than does a person whose life-style does not include these characteristics.

The principles of the wholeness and unity of the person, and of the *uniqueness* of each person, principles that underlie the field of holistic medicine, are well illustrated by Cheraskin's remarks.

The following case history is that of a woman with long-term symptoms that did not lead to a definitive diagnosis.

E. was a married woman in her late twenties. She worked as a secretary in a large company in what she described as "dull work in a dreary office." There were no children.

For about a year and a half she had had a condition of enlarged glands in her neck, armpit, and groin. Repeated medical examinations had ruled out all the usual causes of such a condition, but had been unable to suggest a diagnosis.

A friend recommended a holistic health center, and she decided to try once more to find out what the condition was. The center did a complete medical work-up of its own, but like the other studies this led to no definite diagnosis. The senior counselor at the center then suggested that the appropriate step would be a general upgrading of her life. In this process the condition might disappear. If it did not, at least she would be in a much better position to deal with whatever diagnosis was finally established. E. thought about this suggestion and decided to go ahead with it. She held a series of ten sessions with a health specialist, exploring the different domains of her existence, personal relationships, job and creativity satisfactions, her relations to her body, her relations to her spiritual needs.

Her personal relationships seemed to be in excellent shape. She had a fulfilling marriage, close and warm friends, and good relationships with most family members.

Job satisfactions were zero and there appeared to be little outlet for her intellectual and creative needs. In the course of the discussion she decided to start working toward a master's degree in social work (she had an undergraduate degree in sociology). She decided to go to school for a year at night and then, finances permitting, to go at least half time. She started school in the evening at the beginning of the following semester.

In the physical realm, exploration revealed that she was about thirty pounds overweight, had a diet consisting mostly of junk foods, smoked a pack of cigarettes a day, and took practically no exercise. It was decided that this realm was the first priority on her agenda. A vacation for her and her husband was coming up and they decided to spend it in a way that would put her right to work in this realm. They chose to go to the yoga camp on Paradise Island in the Bahamas. This nonprofit camp, run by a Hindu mystical development group (the Devananda Foundation) serves only organic vegetarian food and the program includes four hours of hatha-yoga a day plus three additional hours of chanting and meditating. For E., as for many others, it was an ideal place to start her program. As no cigarettes are permitted at the camp, she quit "cold turkey" on arrival and found to her surprise that with such a drastic change in life-style, she hardly missed them. By the time she returned home two weeks later, the worst was over and she had not returned to smoking. The diet at the camp left her ten pounds lighter without the feeling of having deprived herself. Since then she has been more careful in her diet although she has not stayed rigidly on the camp food program. She has pretty much given up junk foods, has maintained an essentially vegetarian diet, has added vitamin and mineral supplements, and she has lost another ten pounds.

The hatha-yoga program was one she found that she enjoyed. This modality consists of a series of exercises performed lying, sitting, and standing: a set of positions into which the person moves his body as far as he is able without strain. For each position (asana) there is a counterposition. Thus a forward-bending series of postures is followed by a backward-bending series, and so forth. Each class includes a number of yoga breathing exercises (pranayamas) during which deep relaxation is taught. There is a meditative aspect to hatha-yoga revealed in the attitudes toward the self, the body, and movement that emerge during the teaching. It is certainly one of the finest systems ever devised for tuning the entire body.

E. felt that hatha-yoga, as she learned it from the expert teachers at the camp, was a good way for her to work with her body. Since it is a system that a person can apply on his or her own, she has kept up with it by practicing three times a week for an hour and a half. Once every two weeks or so she attends a class taught by a teacher in her neighborhood in order to make sure that she is doing the asanas correctly and to learn new ones.

On evaluating the spiritual realm of her being, she found it also to be undernourished. In the late sixties and early seventies she had been involved in the antiwar cause and had participated in the Washington marches and similar activities. She had been somewhat involved in the ecology movement, but had never taken an active role. Shortly after her return from the yoga camp, she joined Greenpeace, a very dedicated and effective ecology organization, and began to take an active role in its work. She also began to meditate for twenty minutes a day using the Jesus Prayer (Lord Jesus Christ have mercy on me) as a mantra. This is probably the most extensively used mantra in the world and is used particularly widely in the Eastern Orthodox Church.

Some three to four months after she returned from the yoga camp, her swollen glands began to soften and reduce in size, and by the end of six to seven months they had returned to normal and have not swollen again in the three years since. No diagnosis has ever been established. Her internist has summed up the matter by saying: "Whatever it is you had, you don't have it now." It is entirely possible that the glands would have returned to normal without the program she embarked on, but she feels that even if this were so, the program was well worthwhile. She feels more energy, zest, and mental alertness than she ever recalls having felt before. She rates her life as "very fulfilling."

A postscript to this case may be of interest. After she completed her M.S.W. degree, she and her husband decided that before she began her new career, they would like to start a family. When she was five months pregnant, she slipped on a step and broke her ankle in several places. It was set at the local hospital and there was a good deal of pain in the weeks following. Not wanting to take drugs because of the effect that they might have on the fetus, she began to work with a homeopathic physician. He prescribed arnica (European daisy) immensely diluted (the "shadow of the shadow" of arnica). This eased the pain almost completely.

Homeopathy was developed by Samuel Hahnemann in the early 1800s. A widely respected physician, Hahnemann began to question the very essence of modern medicine by challenging the doctrine of opposites. He introduced the idea that a substance that would cure a disease in an ill person was the same substance that would produce the symptoms in a healthy person. Thus, quinine, which is a specific for malaria, will produce chills and fever (the symptoms of malaria) if given to a healthy person. In his *Organon of the Art of Healing*, he wrote: "... The rule accepted in conventional allopathic medicine to cure by contraries is entirely wrong, and ... to the contrary, diseases vanish and are cured only by medicines capable of producing a similar affection." He found, in opposition to the conventional view, that the more diluted his medicines were, the better they worked. He believed that the smaller the amount of an active ingredient present, the more effective it is, and the fewer side-effects there are.

Although homeopathy is, in theory, directly opposed to some of the most basic concepts of mainline medicine, it must be taken, today, as a serious modality. In the United States, only licensed physicians (M.D.'s and O.D.'s) are legally allowed to practice homeopathy.

I have mentioned several times in this book the new phenomenon of holistic health centers, which are beginning to spring up all over the country. A number of the individuals in the case histories have used them. These centers are of all types. How can a person evaluate them? If you decide to use one, how can you tell if it is really what it claims to be or if it is just the brainstorm of a group of predators or ignoramuses who have decided to cash in on the new trend and have put together a pretty package with no nourishment in it?

(That this is a major tendency in American business should not be forgotten when you're evaluating organizations in the disease and health fields. Just a few years ago, an experiment was described before the McGovern Select Committee on Human Needs. One group of rats was fed one of the new popular breakfast cereals. A control group was fed the ground-up boxes that the cereals came in. The rats that were fed the boxes lived significantly longer than the rats that were fed the cereal.)

In evaluating the package and the contents of a holistic health center, the following concepts should be held in mind.

1. Does the center follow the four basic axioms of holistic medicine? Are you treated as an individual existing on many levels, in many domains, all of equal importance? (Although one must start by dealing with one specific domain, which varies according to the particular problem and the total situation.) Are you met as a unique individual with a program specifically designed for you? Are you actively encouraged to be a full partner in the decision-making process? Are you seen as a person with (at least potentially) strong self-healing and self-repair abilities?

2. The place should be run in a professional manner. I do not mean here that every man has to wear a tie (or a white coat) and every woman a tailored dress or medical whites. I do mean that records should be responsibly maintained, that appointments should be well organized and punctually kept, and that the place should be clean. Among other things, it should be certified by the board of health.

The staff certainly should have professional training. It is essential that there be a qualified physician fully on board. (One on the letterhead and present in the flesh every third Thursday from 11:00 A.M. to 12:00 noon is not enough.) He or she must be part of the team. A nutritionist should have at least a master's degree in nutrition or human physiology, plus supervised experience, and not be someone who has been "interested in the field for a long time and listens regularly to Carleton Fredericks." Social workers and psychologists also should have master's degrees and either be members of the National Association of Social Workers or the American Psychological Association. They should also have had supervised experience and some psychotherapy of their own. Psychiatrists should be at least Board eligible, if not Board certified. If someone there does Rolfing, he or she should be on the approved list of the Ida Rolf Foundation. (Rolfing is a method of very deep, and sometimes painful, massage in which the "Rolfer" manipulates the body in order to return it to a normal and healthy structural and postural position. It is a strenuous technique for freeing the body, mind, and emotions from their negative conditioning. Energies locked in "armoring," the permanent tension of large muscle groups, are freed for living, and this release is accompanied by insight into the anxieties that produced the body armoring. Developed by Ida Rolf in the 1930s, it is also known as Structural Processing or Structural Dynamics.)

Always check the training of anyone you are dealing with in a holistic health center. If the person becomes upset or resentful about this, leave immediately. After all, you must remember that in the view of holistic medicine each domain of your being is as important as all of the others, and must be treated with the same respect. If you wouldn't care to have your head operated on by a surgeon who had read a book entitled *Brain Surgery for Fun and Profit*, and "thought he would like to get into it and watched a lot of operations," then don't let an acupuncturist with somewhat similar qualifications work on you, either.

3. Is there one supervising person working with and helping you make decisions? Unless you are clear as to who the primary health specialist is (working, of course, with the aid of other specialists), you are going to feel fragmented and will wind up trying to work with a number of people with different viewpoints and emphases. There must be one person who is, and stays, in charge of your "case" and who, with you, reaches final decisions.

4. Remember that although the workman is worthy of his hire and that running a center does cost money, an organization devoted to profit will see it as legitimate to exploit you for everything you have. If you have any sense that a center is trying to sell you expensive tests, consultations, and programs rather than trying with you to come to the best possible growth-route to your health, leave the premises. Are they business oriented or service oriented? If the first, this is not a holistic health center, but a racket. Ask if

they have a meaningful sliding schedule of fees or if they perform some free community services. If neither of these, get out. They are business oriented.

The following case is that of a woman with a severe disease who worked as her own health specialist.

S., a woman in her late forties, had achieved a very high position in public relations. She disliked her work, but felt that it was impossible to give up such success. Her marriage was, as she described it, "friendly," but there was little love or warmth in it. It was a routine relationship between two people who had learned to "accommodate" to each other, but that was about all. There were no children.

Abdominal symptoms brought her to a medical examination, at which a stomach cancer with metastases was diagnosed. A chemotherapy program was recommended, but with little optimism. The prognosis was seen as poor. Her husband was told to expect that she would have a fairly rapid decline and would probably die within eighteen months.

Her husband, who did respect his wife as an adult, listened to her plea that she wanted *all* the truth, and told her exactly what the oncologist had told him. She then decided that the medical program as outlined did not hold enough promise to be worth undertaking, particularly as the side effects of the chemotherapy were likely to be very severe.

She determined to design her own program from whatever sources were available and began first to investigate alternative cancer treatments. She decided that since she did not have the training to evaluate the biochemical and cellular aspects of the various treatment programs, she would use her years of experience in business to evaluate the person in charge of each one. She met and talked to about a dozen physicians who were using alternative methods and chose the one who seemed to her to be of the highest personal caliber. She found that they all seemed to make about the same claims for success and that personality was the only indicator that she felt competent to use.

She regarded her medical treatment as the cornerstone of her approach to the cancer, but felt that it was far from sufficient. She began to investigate other domains of her being. She started with a nutrition program that made sense to her and that her physician assured her was not contraindicated by the medical treatment. (He also assured her that it was useless and would not do her any good, but she ignored this as he had had absolutely no training in the field.) Investigating exercise and movement programs, she was unable to follow her first choice—folk dancing—because of her illness, but she found a great deal of enjoyment in a thrice-weekly sensory-awareness (Grindler method) class. She began to feel more at home in her body and more related to it than she had ever felt before in her life. She began to study a form of meditation and meditated twice a day for twenty minutes each time. She started psychotherapy with a therapist whose orientation was on helping her patients find out what was "right" for them (in what ways of being, relating, and creating they would find the fullest joy, zest, and serenity) and what was blocking their expression, rather than on finding out what was "wrong" with them. As a result of the therapy, she decided that a large paycheck and a lot of prestige were not enough return for spending forty of her best hours each week at a job she hated. She resigned (to the horror and disapproval of all her friends and family) and started a new career (in real estate), which she thoroughly enjoyed. She found that rather than dreading each new day, she was glad to get up every morning to go to the office. She was earning far less than before, had no more lunches at fancy restaurants paid for by the company, but was enjoying her life much more.

As she began to grow and change, she insisted that her husband also change. After some badgering, he also started in psychotherapy. As they both grew emotionally, they discovered that they liked each other more. (Their relationship could, of course, as easily have gone the other way and ended in divorce.) The marriage improved considerably, and for the first time became alive and vital.

The year after the woman started the medical program, her tumors regressed. Six years later she is now symptom free and X-rays show no sign of cancer.

It is, of course, entirely possible that she would have responded to the medical treatment without the work on other levels. She even might have responded to the original chemotherapy program as outlined so pessimistically by her first oncologist. We simply cannot know. What she did, however, was to maximize her chances of responding positively. She approached the problem on as many levels of her being as possible and thereby made it much more likely that her self-healing abilities would be fully mobilized. She also improved the general quality of her life to a very considerable extent and certainly made it worth living for whatever time she did have.

By taking her destiny into her own hands and designing a unique and individual program for herself on as many levels as possible, she had followed exactly what we would say today is the basic viewpoint of holistic medicine.

Sensory awareness, the adjunctive modality that S. used in the body sphere, is a method of becoming *aware* of ourselves through physical sensations. In lying, sitting, standing, or during very slow movements, the participant tries to become as conscious as possible of the sensations of the body. There is a deep total and gentle concentration on what is going on in the body and in the breathing. One begins to understand how much one has separated oneself from the body, and the parts of the body from each other. There is a realization that the lack of attention to bodily sensations is an aspect of the fragmentation of the self, and how far this has progressed. One generally leaves a session feeling far different (and much better) physically and emotionally than he did when he entered. The instructor suggests what part of the body to focus the attention on. As one heals the splits within the self, the gulfs between the self and others and the self and the general nature of which we are all a part tend to lessen. It is a Western form of hatha (physical) yoga which was developed in the 1920s in Germany by Elsie Grindler. The best-known teachers of this method today are Charlotte Selver and Corolla Speads.

The form of meditation S. used is one widely used today. It involves the use of a mantra, a very old meditation method in which the individual, as physically relaxed as possible, repeats over and over to himself a chosen phrase. Each time the mind wanders it is gently brought back to the repetition. The classical explanation for the effectiveness of this method is that the carefully chosen phrase has a positive effect on the individual it was chosen for. More modern theory suggests that it is the doing of just one thing at a time, involving as much of the being as possible in a deliberately chosen single activity, that has the desired effect. Thus, some researchers have suggested that any simple (preferably meaningless) word or phrase will do.

In any case, if this meditation is conscientiously done twice a day for twenty minutes at a time, it certainly tends to have positive effects on the meditator. Greater feelings of calmness and ability to cope, a normalization of such variables as blood pressure and blood acid-alkalinity levels, have been widely reported.

There are also a growing number of health specialists who do not work in an organizational setting. The last case in this series is quoted directly from the files of one of these.

Marilyn Ruben of Miami Beach is one of the new health specialists working to define the profession. She calls her work "Catalytic Counseling in Whole Person Health" and defines herself as an "adjunctive professional."

MR. E.: AGE EIGHTY-FOUR YEARS
Personal Data

Independent, though sometimes hesitant or indecisive about making decisions since lost sounding board with death of second wife. Retired at sixty-five from long-term employment with national corporation. Worked most of his life for one employer as bookkeeper/accountant. Has continued lifelong habit of self-education, attending college-level courses sponsored by employer over the years and through avid reading on many subjects.

Continues "making the best of each day," taking one day at a time, grateful for both mental and physical capacities allowing him to continue "to enjoy my life." Is very aware that his physical capacities and mental faculties at eighty-four years of age set him apart from many younger persons with chronic and often severe problems. Mr. E. often "feels like a dinosaur. Most people my age are dead or in a nursing home." Since wife's death, has taken over care of senile sister, administering trust income for her maximum benefit and comfort; and says doing that "gives me something to do and someone to care for."

"Something to do" includes what has now come to be a weekly routine of errands, cooking his breakfast and supper, visiting sister twice weekly, going five days a week to spa for morning period of "working out" in gym and pool, attending the local school hot-lunch program afterward for well-balanced, nutritious meal, as well as socializing with neighborhood friends, working in the garden—doing all but heaviest work—housecleaning (vacuuming, mopping, dusting), and weekly laundry. Add to that, maintains and operates own car (is good driver), supervises repairs on house when necessary, and goes out to restaurants alone or with friends, though prefers not to drive at night. Thus, "I don't know where the time goes."

Recent Past Medical History

Intermittent periods of high blood pressure or lowered heart rate/poor circulation brought on by worry about, as well as deliberate difficult situations provoked by, semisenile sister.

Chronic gout in one or the other foot requiring periodic

review by physician. Degenerative osteoarthritis of right hip and lower spine causing pain and difficulty in walking and sitting.

Sinus headaches with possible migraine developing if pressured emotionally by sister's efforts to create turmoil. Liver enlarged from prolonged use of heavy liquor (which no longer drinks). Recent corrective prostate surgery, minor procedure, approximately two years ago. Successful cataract surgery on right eye approximately ten years ago.

Present Illness
Some chronic problems as outlined in recent past medical history. Varying degrees of depression from mild to severe from period of wife's death in 1974 through mid-1980.

History of Professional Intervention to Create
Individual Program for "Whole Person Health"
Prior to Mr. E.'s decision to follow through with necessary corrective prostate surgery, we had held weekly discussions regarding the ongoing maintenance possibilities of improving various health factors and continuing said maintenance upon health improvement as a way to increase the quality of life. Included was a careful review of low-salt- and low-purine-content diet (copies were given to Mr. E.) to be supplemented with vitamins and certain minerals; a review of medication and management which turned up a severe depressive reaction to Valium prescribed for sleeping, resulting in its elimination and the temporary substitution of meprobamate in its place. Mr. E. was further advised to avoid tyramine-rich foods when taking Aldoril for hypertension; and information was included regarding the relationship of hypertension to adequate fluid volume intake and the use of salicylates. He was advised to eliminate high protein or acidic substances that reduce the effectiveness of Benemid and Colchecine, which was used in treatment of his gout.

Before the above recommendations were made, Mr. E. was being treated for hypertension and gout with two drugs in direct opposition to each other. The undesirable side effects were immediate, luckily none permanently damaging. (Mr. E. did not return to prescribing physician.) With confidence in a new internist, and with a surgeon available through his medical insurance program, Mr. E. underwent prostate surgery with no ill effects, recovering fully in the projected time of four or five weeks. Through an insurance company error, his surgery was covered; but he was no longer eligible to receive further medical care because the policy had ceased with wife's death. This precipitated an uneasy period of not having medical supervision for about six months until Mr. E. contacted an internist in his neighborhood who told him everything was fine (although Mr. E. knew the gouty condition was not under control) and recommended that he "come back and see me in three months." Mr. E. said, "At my age, hell, in three months I could be dead," and made a decision to find more concerned medical care. Mr. E. was referred by me to Dr. Harold H. Bloomfield, Center for Holistic Medicine in California. Mr. E. has found there a physician in whom he has trust and confidence; and most importantly, a physician who respects and understands Mr. E.'s wish to play intelligently a large part in his health management. Since this physician also understands the effectiveness of my professional intervention, he has willingly checked my recommendations for validity as they have come up in discussion weekly with Mr. E. These have been the suggested possibility of acupuncture for arthritis in his hip and spine when needed; a check for possible allergy as related to sinus headache after review of family history; thorough exam and CAT scan to make sure no other possibilities existed (Chlor-Trimeton was prescribed, resulting in some relief); and as blood pressure is now more reasonably within normal limits, the daily dosage of Aldoril has been lowered.

Discussions of stress management and relaxation techniques have pinpointed a long-established habit of physical labor in the garden to resolve physical tension and ease the mind "in admiring the beautiful flowers I grow," a technique serving an effective purpose, I believe, just as other methods more formally taught.

We have ranged far and wide in discussion of religion and philosophy: Mr. E.'s personal philosophy of death without fear as well as the full enjoyment of life, matters relating to a will, and the setting up and implementation of a trust to care for his sister in the event of his death or disability from illness.

Mr. E. has underscored the fact that at his age, with his wife gone, no children, and his sister incapacitated, much of his need for in-depth communication has been fulfilled through our working together.

Results

Through actively managing own diet and medication, through implementation of an exercise program which he himself has worked out benefiting oxygen intake and improving leg circulation, and through an occasional series of acupuncture treatments when necessary, Mr. E. is able to walk at a steady pace with good balance and sit without pain and discomfort. His appetite is good and he no longer requires medication for sleep. With a firm and well-muscled body, Mr. E. stands tall and erect, looking fifteen to twenty years younger than actual age of eighty-four.

Mentally alert, he has an active continuing interest in local and world politics, sports of all kinds, gardening and horticulture, travel, archaeology, as well as the many other subjects that have intrigued him over the years, and is "still delighted at the sight of a pretty woman."

His latest comment was, "Been feeling pretty good. It's been a good week. Don't know what happened but I'm not complaining." (Laughter.) With trust set up and function-

ing, will in order, and other details arranged in an orderly
fashion in the event of his death, Mr. E. has set about to enjoy life even more fully, and with his medical advisor's permission, celebrates the close of each day with two glasses
of wine.

The adjunctive modality of acupuncture which Mr. E. used
is a very old Chinese method of treating disease. The theory
behind it concerns hypothetical flows of energy along certain body paths ("meridians") and the concept that these
paths of vital energy sometimes go out of equilibrium, causing disease. Balance and equilibrium of these flows can be
restored by the expert through a process of inserting the
tips of fine needles under the skin in exactly the right
places. The number of needle points that are inserted, the
depth of penetration, and the length of time that they are
left in depends on the condition being treated. The process
is almost painless and helps a wide variety of conditions.

The cases presented here may lead to a false conclusion,
as all of them resulted in successful resolutions of the presenting problem. I have chosen these specific cases because
they are the clearest examples that I could find of the state
of the art in a rapidly developing field, but holistic medicine
does not always work this well. I know of a number of individuals with cancer, multiple sclerosis, heart conditions,
and the like, who used holistic techniques and still died of
their disease. Nearly all felt that the attempt was worthwhile
and that it had enabled them to get the most out of their
lives.

Nothing works 100 percent of the time. All systems
limp, all techniques sometimes fail. Further, we are a mortal
race and will, each and every one of us, die of our mortality.
At our birth, we incur a debt to death and it will be called.

The holistic approach makes no guarantees. What it
does do is maximize the chances that our self-healing re-

sources will be effective. It brings our own resources to the aid of mainline medical programs. All medical programs have three classes of response from those who participate in them: "poor," "average," "excellent." Holistic medicine helps us improve the statistical chance that we will be in the highest class. Along the way, it also insures that we get as much as is possible out of ourselves and our lives.

Physicians and homeopaths, nutritionists and Tai-chi teachers, psychotherapists and psychic healers, we all die. However, we can live our lives to the fullest—physically, mentally, and spiritually. This is what the holistic approach is all about.

HOW TO SURVIVE IN A HOSPITAL

Overheard in a hospital corridor:

FIRST WOMAN: The doctor said she should take the medicine regularly.
SECOND WOMAN: Doctors, what do they care?

A long-term hospital patient was asked: "How do you like the people in this hospital?" He replied, "There are no people here. There are only doctors, nurses, and patients."

These two true incidents have in their implications a strange grain of truth. When you enter a hospital, you are entering a new world. If you understand this, you will know better how to behave and how to achieve the maximum possible benefits from your stay. You will also know how to avoid the special pitfalls and dangers implicit in being a hospital patient.

First you must understand what a hospital *is*. It is a business organization, in the last analysis run by accountants, which sells certain tests, remedies, and procedures related to disease. It is staffed by people who came into the field generally from the best of motives. They were given a medical education, and are in a medical system oriented to viewing the patient not as a person but as a broken machine. They work in a milieu that reinforces this orientation by ghettoizing the patients, segregating them by disease or by dysfunctioning organ system. Since the staff

182

stays in the hospital and patients come and go, they eventually begin more and more to see the hospital procedures as something that should be designed for their own comfort and convenience rather than for the patients'. Patients in pain, anguish, and fear constantly pressure them to behave in omniscient and omnipotent ways. Little by little they begin to act as if they could fill these roles, and train younger colleagues also to act in this way. Presently they begin to believe that these are their proper roles and become upset when challenged.

Doctors are so completely oriented to fighting disease and ignoring the person who has it that, in catastrophic illness, they often seem to be asking themselves: "How many heroic measures and mutilating operations can be charged to the patient (or to the insurance company) before death—the final method of consumer resistance—is allowed to intervene?"

They define a "good" patient as one who accepts their statements and their actions uncritically and unquestioningly. A "bad" patient is one who asks questions to which they do not have the answers, raises problems they are uncomfortable with, and does not accept hospital procedures as necessarily wise, useful, or intelligent. There is a tremendous pressure on the staff to regard the institution's rules as correct and the individual patient who objects to them as wrong. In spite of all these pressures, an amazingly large minority of the staff at most hospitals care about their patients and regard them as individuals. A majority succumb to a greater or lesser degree to the pressures and become institution- rather than patient-oriented.

The high cost of medical care arises in large part from duplication of services among neighboring hospitals, which is largely due to competition for prestige (and profits). If patient care were the major concern, it would be easy for the boards of directors of hospitals in the same area to come to an agreement as to which hospitals should specialize in which services. As specialized equipment and facilities are becoming increasingly technological and expensive, this kind of agreement would save a great deal of money. However, given a realistic view of the present situation, asking hospitals to do this is roughly the equivalent of asking Ford and General Motors to agree as to which one will make small cars and which one will make station wagons.

It is very difficult for even the most dedicated physician or nurse to maintain a service orientation while working in an institution devoted to profit making. It soon becomes clear to all employees that the product of their organization is tests and medical procedures, not patient care. To retain the attitude that "the care of the patient comes first" is very difficult when the entire hospital has another attitude entirely. The really amazing thing about the modern hospital is that there are so many caring people working in it, and that the patient care is as good as it is.

If you recognize that the hospital is a business selling a product and that it is part (with the insurance companies and the pharmaceutical houses) of one of the largest and most lucrative industries in America, you will not be too surprised at some of the incidents of complete "uncaring" that you will probably encounter in any reasonably long stay in a hospital. Within just a few weeks' time, the author has personally seen the following:

1. A postsurgical patient was returned to his bed, but his nurse's bell was not attached. He was the only patient in a multiple-bed room. He did not see anyone for a period of six hours after being returned to his bed. Part of this time he was in severe pain and unable to summon help.
2. A patient, unable to move himself, was left on a bedpan for two and a half hours. No one answered his bell-pull, and his back muscles became knotted in pain. Finally, another patient passing in the hall

heard him weeping, asked him what the problem was, and then went to the nurses' station at the end of the hall, where he convinced a nurse's aide that she ought to respond to the patient's agony.

3. A patient who had returned from major abdominal surgery two days before had just had her catheter removed after voiding a large quantity of urine. She was now, an hour later, in extreme pain, her muscles spasming and threatening to tear open her incision. The patient complained that she had to void more urine. For over an hour three different nurses told her that she was hysterical. She was given tranquilizers and told that she was making a nuisance of herself, and that there were patients who had *real* pain and needed the nurses' attention. Suddenly, in the midst of her crying it became apparent that she was wetting the bed. The nurses looked at the wet sheets and decided to put the catheter back. When it was in, she voided 700 cc. of urine (that's a lot) through it. Not one of the nurses apologized or indicated in any way that they had been brutalizing the patient.

It would be possible to mention a myriad of personally witnessed incidents of this kind, but those mentioned give a sense of what may well happen during any hospital stay. I should add that these three incidents happened to intelligent, middle-class patients in hospitals with international reputations. It is because of incidents such as these, as well as other more serious mistakes that can have long-range effects, that you need to know how to defend yourself in a hospital.

During the same period of time that I saw these unfortunate events, I saw a much larger number of examples of caring, protective, and life-saving behavior.

When you enter a hospital for a procedure or set of procedures, you are immediately subject to a routine whose effect is to strip you of all signs and symbols of your autonomous adult status and make you into a passive, dependent, childlike person who will not question or oppose those in authority. You can no longer decide what you will wear or eat, or go anywhere alone (often not even to the bathroom). Strangers take complete authority over your life and destiny, order you to wake up, go to sleep, turn over to be examined or washed, and generally act as if you are a not-too-bright child and they are adults.

The hospital patient is made to follow passively a routine, which he is prevented from comprehending by a strange and esoteric language and by the attitude that he simply does not have the training or knowledge to understand what is happening. He is quickly made to feel that a "good patient" behaves in the same way as a good and obedient child, who does as he is told, never asks difficult questions, and agrees that everything is fine as long as the adults are in charge (no matter what the actual situation is).

A friend of mine, whom I admire greatly, was hospitalized after a heart attack. While in the cardiac care unit, she was attached to a machine that monitored her heart. Suddenly the machine stopped clicking away. A nurse came galloping into the room and was about to do various dramatic things to start my friend's heart pumping again, when my friend pointed out sharply that she was sitting up in bed, drinking some orange juice, and was very much alive. The nurse shouted, "But you *can't* be! Your heart has stopped beating!" My friend suggested that maybe the *machine* was the problem, an idea that seemed to strike the nurse as ridiculous. But shortly thereafter an electrician arrived on the scene.

I think my friend's story is a realistic metaphor for what life is like in many hospitals these days. There are exceptions, thank heavens, but the age of technology has turned some hospitals into machine shops in which very advanced and life-saving equipment is looked upon with awe, while people are considered an incidental inconvenience.

When you are desperately ill and realize that doctors and machinery and hospital care may well make the difference between life and death, your own judgment and your sense of personal identity are often impaired. Think how many weak and sick and frightened patients there are who might almost have been convinced that they *were* dead when the machine stopped working!

Edgar Jackson, probably the world's outstanding specialist in crisis management, describes very well, in his excellent and important *Coping with the Crisis of Your Life*, what happens when one becomes a hospital patient. Even a professional who knows the hospital procedures and routines is quickly and expertly reduced from an independent adult to a passive child.

> From that moment on, I was no longer the person I had been. Instead, I was a pliable, compliant inhabitant of a world of vague feelings and limited comprehension. I had been delivered, body, mind, and spirit, into the hands of my physicians. I was a completely dependent and defenseless creature surrounded by those who exerted authority over me.

Doctors often defend the process of patient infantilization by insisting that it is necessary for the smooth running of the hospital, is what is wanted by the patients, and, in fact, is good for them. The infantilization is, of course, simply for the convenience and emotional comfort of the staff, not the patients, and is a product of the basic belief that people who are sick are like machines that are broken. They don't work (i.e., can't function as adults), and therefore must be fixed by a mechanic. Naturally, the machine sits there completely passively while the mechanic does all the work. The staff has been trained to deal with diseases and not with people. And this is what they do.

Max Parrott, president of the American Medical Association, wrote:

> It has often been said that the technical aspects of medicine are easy. The difficult part is dealing with the personality of the patient, the so-called psychological or human factor. This takes up a great deal of the time of the practicing physician. It is harder on the doctor's constitution than all of the technical aspects of medicine. It may even cause his or her demise, in the case of a physician with an autonomic nervous system that can't take the heat.

Some years ago, I instituted a program in a hospital with many long-term patients. An hour after each patient was admitted, a volunteer wheeled into the patient's room a cart containing a hundred good-sized reproductions of famous paintings. The reproductions were professionally mounted on light beaverboard and the patient was invited to make a selection and decorate his or her room. The volunteer returned once a week to ask the patient if he or she wanted to exchange the prints for others. The program cost the hospital nothing, except for the time of one volunteer. (The paintings were donated by an art company to which I had explained the purpose.) The program was instituted against the strong opposition of most of the staff. The only objection verbalized was that the program "would cause confusion." The unspoken objection was that it gave the patients a sense of individuality, of being persons with a disease, rather than being a disease with a person somehow attached to it, and that it treated the patients as adults. The patient response to the program was very strong and positive and the program continued very successfully for the next two years. Within three months of my leaving the hospital for another job, the program was discontinued.

Another example would be the experience of anyone

who has battled with hospital personnel to establish a simple rule: that nonmedical personnel such as floor sweepers, newspaper sellers, and so forth, should be required to knock at a closed hospital room door (behind which someone might well be sitting on a bedpan) before entering the room. The fierce and emotional opposition of the staff to such a rule reveals their basic attitude that the patient is no longer an individual human being worthy of respect.

We know from long experience that individualizing patients and expanding their sense of themselves as individuals and adults serves to mobilize their self-healing abilities and bring them to the aid of the medical program. (Every experienced oncologist knows, for example, that "bad patients" tend to survive longer and to respond better to medical intervention than do "good patients.") However, next to the basic orientation that sick patients should be seen only in terms of their disease and that all results are up to the formal medical intervention and not to the individual's self-healing powers, this information is ignored and the antitherapeutic routine of the average hospital weakens the patient's ability to fight for his own recovery.

The concept of self-defense and self-repair is a central contribution of holistic medicine. The idea—not new to medicine, but one which has, in this century, played only a minor role—is that if given a positive environment—socially, emotionally, nutritionally, spiritually—the body's self-healing abilities can do a great deal. This is in accord with the famous statement of the great physician Harvey Cushing: "The task of the physician is to protect the patient from the patient's relatives so that nature can heal him." We are just beginning to appreciate the wisdom behind the wit of this statement, and to find out all the things we have to protect the patient from. Sadly, these often include our own medical techniques.

When you enter a hospital, it is important for you, or someone with you, to understand the medical situation.

You have left the private relationship with your physician and entered a large organization devoted to selling a product and making a profit. Although the hospital is staffed by many people, most of them caring and concerned about you, the overall organization is dedicated—as are *all* organizations—primarily to perpetuating its own existence and growth.

For this new situation you need to prepare a plan.

First, particularly if the procedures are going to be strenuous or will include surgery, if possible have a friend or relative who can be your advocate. Preferably this person should be someone who is not likely to be easily overawed and is not afraid to make a fuss and to ask difficult questions. Not being cut off from the outside world, not being stressed by pain, illness, or surgical procedures, this advocate can represent you when and if you are unable to represent yourself. By and large, the more interest your relatives or advocate shows in your health, the better hospital care you will get.

A few years ago, I was visiting a close relative in one of Manhattan's finest hospitals. She was in a double room and the woman in the next bed was in her late seventies, very weak, and obviously malnourished. Each time I saw her, she seemed thinner and more like a refugee from a Nazi concentration camp. One day I saw her lunch tray being picked up and returned to the cart after lunch. The tray was untouched. She had eaten nothing. I made it my business to be there at supper the following day. The same thing happened. Her tray was brought to her, set on the bed table in front of her, and an hour later was picked up and taken away. She was too weak and malnourished to eat.

Deciding to be her advocate, I went to the charge nurse on the floor and reported the situation. She promised to take care of it. However, at lunch the next day nothing had changed. I then went downstairs to the nurse supervisor's office and again fully reported the story. By that evening, there was dramatic improvement. A nurse's aide had been assigned to the woman at each meal. The patient quickly started to gain weight and strength and by the time my relative left the hospital, she was eating by herself, walking up and down the corridor, and was at least ten pounds heavier.

If I had known her physician, I would certainly have reported the problem to him before telling the charge nurse. If I had had no success with the nurse supervisor's office, I would have gone to the office of the administrative director. For personal care the chain of complaint is: charge nurse, nurse supervisor, hospital administrator, hospital director.

Once you have an advocate, your next priority is information. Before you enter the hospital, there are certain facts you should have and certain questions you should ask.

1. Who is the physician in overall charge of you? Make sure that there is someone who is running the show who has an overview of you and the problem that brought you to the hospital. Ideally that person should be your personal physician and, in most cases, it will be. But be certain that this is the case and find out how often you will see him or her before you enter the hospital.

   Unless there is a coordinating physician, very often in the modern hospital a diagnosis is made according to the specialty of the diagnostician rather than to the illness of the patient. For example, a patient who sees a psychiatrist may receive a diagnosis of "psychosomatic gastrointestinal disorder," while if he sees an internist, the diagnosis may be "pylorospasm." In one case the problem is seen as in his mind, in the other case in his gut. In neither case is there likely to be a multilevel approach to treating the entire person and the many contributing factors to the disease.

2. What is the diagnosis, and how certain of it is your physician?

3. What is the usual course of the disease, both without therapy and with therapy?
4. What are the side effects of the therapy?
5. What alternatives exist?

When diagnostic tests are prescribed, you will want to know how painful they will be, what side effects they will have, and—most importantly—whether they will make a real difference (a "real difference" is a difference that makes a difference). Will the physician's course of action change depending on the results of the test? *If not, there is no reason to take it.* There is an increasing tendency to give more and more tests. Between 1967 and 1972, for example, there was an increase of 33 percent in the number of laboratory tests conducted per hospital admission. There was no corresponding increase in medical knowledge during that period.

Remember that the hospital is in the business of selling services and these include diagnostic tests. In addition, no physician or hospital was ever sued for malpractice for making too many tests and being *too* thorough in an examination.

Some medical students were asked why they wanted to do a particular arduous diagnostic procedure on their patient. One of them answered that their chief resident had said that only three things were important in medicine: "The diagnosis, the diagnosis, and the diagnosis." While the story may be apocryphal, it illustrates a common medical attitude, particularly in the idealized setting represented by the university teaching hospital. In a particular patient the search for a diagnosis may acquire a life of its own, and in working toward that diagnosis the patient's original complaints, life situation, needs, fears, and economics may become irrelevant. The scenario is directed more by available technology, the special interests of the [hospital] personnel, the schedules of the institution, and above all, the hidden nature of the disease, which must be found because, like Mount Everest, "it is there."

The more tests that are made, the more likely the results of at least one will look unusual. Tests generate more tests and often unwanted and unnecessary treatments are indicated by test results. We then find ourselves as patients embarked on a medical program we do not need.

The famous Wassermann diagnostic blood test for syphilis has been used for forty years. Only lately have we discovered that it is a hypersensitive test and that about half of the individuals diagnosed as syphilitic by it *did not have the disease!* There are numerous other medical procedures that are more popular than validated.

Frequently there is a deep gap in the communication between patient and physician. They may seem to be communicating and think that they are communicating, but their assumptions are so different that both are bound to be disappointed and angered by their relationship. Often the patient is saying something like:

Make me feel good. Fix my life, which isn't working. This is what I am paying you for.

While the physician is saying something like:

Respect me, since I bring the best of modern science to the treatment of your disease. This is what you are paying me for.

Neither is really aware of his underlying assumptions. Neither is going to be happy about the results.

One study showed that when a physician said to a patient, "You will be going home in a few days," this meant one or two days to a majority of the patients. To a majority of the physicians it meant two to four days. Communication is a fragile thing at best. When you are speaking to a physician about an illness, keep checking to make sure that you are hearing each other. Many problems can be prevented if you take it upon yourself to keep the lines of communication clear. Your advocate may be helpful here.

Do not let yourself be ignored if there is something that the physician should know or should be paying attention to. The word *no* is powerful. Use it and be stubborn in repeating it until you are convinced that your objections have been responded to reasonably. Recently in a large New York hospital a patient was being evaluated. Although it was not urgently indicated, and was not of very high priority in the examination, the physician decided to use a dye test for evaluating kidney function (IVP). The patient told the doctor that she was allergic to the dye, that on a previous examination in another city she had been given the test and that she had had a severe negative reaction. Since this was not in the physician's experience, he did not listen to her and gave her the test anyway. The patient died. A simple but stubborn "No, I will not take the test" would have saved her life. Occasionally, you will also have to shout and throw things to get the hospital staff to pay attention to you as a specific individual. You are very likely, of course, to get angry reactions if you say no to something, but your stand may well save your life.

You must also control the number of people who will give you physical examinations. The resident on your service needs to examine you because if anything goes wrong, he or she has to make quick decisions and so must know your body from direct examination. Ask your personal physician if there are any other physicians who *must* do this. If there are, list them on a pad of paper on your bed table, and refuse anyone else. You are allowed to say no. When you are ill there is no reason you should cooperate in a hospital research project or help an intern build up his or her quota of examinations by doing one on you.

If you feel truly sorry for the intern's hard-luck story about his quota, ask your advocate if he or she minds having a physical examination! This will generally bring the intern up short and add some common sense to the discussion.

If you are a woman, only one person should do a breast examination. Unless you are in a gynecological service, no one should do a pelvic examination, and you do not need a Pap test. If your physician wants to make an exception to these particular rules, he or she should explain the reasons in detail. "Hospital procedure" is not a reason.

On the pad of paper on your bedside table, have your physician list all the medications you are supposed to get, at what times you get each, and *what each one looks like*. If a nurse or aide gives you a medicine that doesn't fit your physician's description, refuse it. Even at the best hospitals, a lot of medications get sent to the wrong people.

Find out what diet you will be on and whether you can have food brought in from the outside. As Hippocrates said, "Food or drink slightly inferior in itself, but more pleasant, should be preferred to that better in itself but less pleasant."

You can, of course, go to either extreme on this. The rule of some nutritionists has been that food should be "good of itself," pure and free from contaminants, even if it tastes like parsnip sprouts in wallpaper glue. The other extreme is that the appetizing quality of food—the way it looks and tastes—should be the critical factor and it does not matter very much if the food is full of the kinds of additives that otherwise are used in the manufacture of tanning materials. In both of these cases there is the implication that some aspects of the human being are of real importance and certain other aspects are not. From the viewpoint of serious holistic medicine, *all* aspects are of real importance, although a healthy specialist may, of necessity, work first with one aspect and later with the others. In regard to food, Hippocrates was clearly suggesting a middle course, in line with our modern viewpoint, with the emphasis slightly on the appealing quality.

The average hospital serves food that is neither appetizing nor nutritious. They have generally managed to produce food that is "inferior in itself"—white bread is usually served along with nearly everything else full of contaminants—and at the same time unappealing and unappetizing. They have managed to combine the worst features of institutional food and junk food. A few hospitals, employing trained chefs and nutritionists, have shown that it is possible to produce attractive and healthful meals.

The most important people involved in your personal care are the nurses. The charge nurse (the chief nurse of your floor) on each of the three shifts will come in to introduce herself and to see you the first day. If she does not, send her a message that you would like to meet her. One of the supervisors of the nursing service will also look in every day or so. The charge nurse and the nursing supervisor are the ones to talk to if there is any problem with personal care. Feel free to complain. You do not have to be a "good" child. Complaints *will* get you better service.

In 1972, the American Hospital Association adopted a series of resolutions for the protection of the patient. These became known as the Patient's Bill of Rights. It is now accepted by all hospitals sanctioned by the JCAH (Joint Commission on Accreditation of Hospitals). The Bill of Rights states in part: "Any competent adult has the absolute right to refuse treatment. Any competent adult has the absolute right to refuse to be examined by any particular individual. Any competent adult has the absolute right to refuse to participate in teaching activities."

You also have the right to know the results of all tests made on you, including your blood pressure and pulse rates. It will make it easier, and save a lot of arguments, if you tell your physician to make a note in your chart and to inform the nursing station that any questions you ask are to be answered. Hospital personnel use all sorts of excuses, but the real reason they tell patients as little as possible ("Hush, dear, everything is fine") is because patients are supposed to be good children who don't ask questions, but do just as they are told.

You also have a right to see your chart anytime you wish. (Most hospital personnel become terribly upset if you ask to do this, but if you consult your lawyer he will bear you out and if necessary remind the hospital that you are an adult, competent human being who retains a lawyer.) There is, however, one problem with this. It may *not* be wise to read your own chart. Very often certain terms have one meaning for the lay person and quite another for those with formal medical training. There may be material in your chart that appears alarming to you, but is not at all alarming to the physician. My advice would be to ask your physician to keep you closely informed of test results and the other material in your chart, but don't try to read the chart yourself. If, however, you cannot get the information verbally, read it.

You can leave the hospital at any time. If anyone prevents you from doing so, you can sue for false imprisonment. The hospital may request you to sign an AMA (against medical advice) form, but they can only request this and cannot hold you if you refuse. Incidentally, the small number of studies that have been done on patients who left hospitals against medical advice show that few patients later regret it, and few experience adverse effects. The main damage done is usually to the sense of omnipotence of the hospital staff.

Unauthorized medical treatments (except in clear and obvious life-or-death situations) constitute assault and battery. It does not matter whether the treatment was advisable or not, successful or not. Consent is the key.

As far as surgical procedures go, the rule is the less the better. Do not allow surgeons to remove organs "because there might be trouble with them later and as long as you're opened up, you might as well eliminate the potential problem. . . ." A large number of women with fibroid cysts of the uterus have had their uterus and ovaries removed on this basis. The surgeons told them that they could always use synthetic hormones. Then it was found that the use of the synthetic hormones tended to produce cancer. That treatment is now unavailable. I know of not a single surgeon who ever expressed any regret over these women or apologized to one of them.

In contemplating the removal of an organ or organs, remember that Nature does not indulge in luxuries. As Galen wrote: "Nature does nothing in vain." If it is there, there is a good reason for it. No substitute is going to be as good. (Mother Nature knows best.) Removal should be done if the alternative *at this time* is completely unacceptable. You can always have it removed later. You can't have it put back.

It seems to have disturbed no one that after recent doctors' and hospital strikes in a number of cities (in some of which only 15 percent of the hospital beds in the city were used) there was no noticeable increase in suffering, and certainly no increase in the mortality statistics. A strike in a factory that reduced its output to 15 percent of normal would certainly lead to a decline in the goods produced. If the product of the hospital is supposed to be a decrease in suffering and a lowering of the death rate, why do we not see evidence of this? Perhaps we have no adequate measure of human suffering. But we do know how many people die each month and of what. Is it possible that there is far more wrong with our medical and hospital system than we've dreamed? Is this why no one has asked if the other 85 percent of the hospital beds are really necessary, or if they are simply connected to a very large business that has lost sight of some of its primary goals—such as caring for the suffering—and now operates largely in terms of profit and loss? Is the reason we do not inquire about these other 85 percent of the hospital beds the same reason that no one asks why General Motors can't start making fewer cars each year?

In 1934, the American Child Health Association studied M.D.s' reports on the advisability of tonsillectomy for 1,000 children: 611 had already had their tonsils removed. The re-

maining 389 were then examined by other physicians and
174 more were selected for tonsillectomy. This left 215 children whose tonsils were apparently normal. Another group
of doctors were put to work examining these 215 children,
and 99 of them were adjudged in need of tonsillectomy.
Still another group of doctors was then employed to examine the remaining children and nearly half were recommended for the operation.

Among the things you should carry with you to the hospital are the usual medications you take regularly or occasionally (such as headache or allergy remedies). Ask your
regular physician *before you enter the hospital* if any of
these are contraindicated by the procedures you will undergo. Then keep your medications in your purse or bedside
table. If someone tries to take them away, you or your advocate friend should simply forbid it. Just because there are
"hospital regulations" doesn't mean you have to obey them.
In addition, particularly if you are to have surgery, bring
some glycerine suppositories. (People are frequently badly
constipated after surgery and many tests. And by many pain
killers. For reasons I don't understand, most hospitals will
only give you a suppository when you are impacted up to
the shoulder blades.)

On the aforementioned pad, have written your personal
physician's professional and home telephone numbers as
well as the name and numbers of any physicians who will
have much to do with you while you are a patient—surgeon, anesthetist, etc. It's wise to look up their telephone
numbers and record them also. Use any and all these numbers if you need to.

Above all, don't be afraid to be difficult when something is wrong. If the sheets are not changed or your medication is not delivered in a reasonable approximation of the
time for which it was ordered, push your nurse's bell and
complain. If you are bleeding and no one answers your
bell—scream. In short, if you are in the hospital for the convenience of the staff, be a "good" patient. If you are there

because you are sick and want to get the maximum benefits from your stay, then do everything possible to retain your adult status and as much control as you can over your own destiny.

If you have pain while in the hospital, do not be heroic about it. Every study shows that people who receive their pain medication when the pain first starts need much less of it and ask for it less often than do people who wait until they can't stand it anymore. The longer you wait, the more muscles in the area are going to tighten up and the more the pain will increase. The more sore and painful the whole area becomes because of muscle spasms, the less effect the pain medication will have and the more likely it is that the pain will quickly return after the medication wears off. Heroism is out of place in hospitals.

If you are not in a hospital, but have to go to a hospital emergency room, it is also most helpful if you can have someone with you. If this person can be a strong advocate who will stay until a decision has been made as to what the problem is and what to do about it, so much the better.

Let us say that it is three o'clock in the morning and you go to the emergency room with severe pain. While you are waiting for the ambulance, if there is no one who can accompany you, try to phone someone to meet you at the hospital. When you arrive, you or your advocate should make a fuss. Tell whoever is in charge loudly and clearly how severe your pain is and that you think you are going to faint. It is true that the meek may inherit the earth, but unless you are in a hurry to inherit your six feet of it, do not be meek. If the nurses or other staff say they are too short of time to treat you now, or if the examining physician does not show up in a reasonable time, pick up a phone and call the administrative director. There is always one on duty. Or better, have your advocate go to his office and make a fuss there.

Presently you will see the examining physician. You or

your advocate should get his or her name. (Physicians, like other people, work better if someone is watching and knows who they are.) In addition you or your advocate should ascertain (either then or, in some cases, in the morning) what examinations were made and what the diagnosis was.

In one of the large metropolitan hospitals in New York City in 1976, there was an impostor physician in the emergency room for several months. With no training, but with the necessary white uniform, he saw patients, ordered tests, and made dispositions until he was accidentally unmasked. This, of course, was an extremely rare occurrence. Follow in the emergency room the same general rules that apply to any hospital stay. Allow no arduous procedure until you understand why it is necessary and what the alternatives are. Be stubborn about this. It is likely to save you discomfort and money; it may save your life.

One last word about emergency rooms. Leave jewelry at home and bring only enough money to pay the required fees. Things have a habit of disappearing in these places.

In the past few pages, I have been writing of the negative aspects of many present-day hospitals and have presented a very unfair and biased picture. I have emphasized these aspects in order to help people protect themselves against them. A more complete picture would take into account the fact that the modern hospital is far superior to any institutions we have had in the past. Hospitals save a vast number of lives and prevent a vast amount of pain. One need only be very ill, or have an ill child, to experience the positive aspects as well. It is entirely legitimate to criticize the modern hospital system strongly so as to try to make it better and to help patients function better within it. It is also more legitimate to thank God that the modern hospital is there when we need it.

CONCLUSIONS

Where do we go from here? The tremendous advances in the ability of modern medicine to intervene successfully in the infectious and contagious diseases have been of inestimable value to mankind, but this very success has impeded our ability to perceive, and to use to the fullest, the other half of the medical process—the patient's self-defense and self-healing abilities. The progress we have made is a great "good." The "best" would be an integration and synthesis of the two. It is this growing awareness, on the part of both the lay public and the medical profession, that is at the heart of the present confusion and ferment in medicine.

Throughout the history of Western civilization, the conflict over which of these two principles the physician should stress has raged back and forth. Should the medical focus be on conquering disease or should it be on helping the patient to strengthen and use his natural resources and grow toward health? With the technological advances of the past century, particularly the development of the germ theory and the alliance of medicine and chemistry, the pendulum has swung to the extreme of active intervention. In recent times the physician has sought to "treat the disease in the body in the bed," to use his new and immense resources to "overcome" the disease, and has largely ignored the patient's self-healing abilities.

The technological viewpoint that has been so

much a part of our culture has further influenced the physician to view the sick person as a broken machine that needs fixing. The goal has been to diagnose and repair, to find out what part is not functioning and why, and fix it. Since a machine does not have self-repair abilities (any more than it has feelings, attitudes, hopes, or fears), these have come to be regarded as less and less important in medical training.

In addition, the mechanical viewpoint and the germ theory reinforced the notion that each disease had one specific cause and, therefore, each disease had one specific treatment. There was supposedly a "correct" treatment for each problem and the very great difference between human individuals was largely forgotten. This idea was so widely accepted that the experience of generations of physicians that people are very different in their vulnerability to disease and in their response to it and to medical treatment was almost forgotten. The warnings of many outstanding medical specialists were ignored.

This approach to disease made great advances possible. It provided a method for virtually wiping out the threat of many killer communicable and infectious diseases. But it has been far less effective in dealing with degenerative diseases.

The successes have appeared to many of us to herald a new era of health. Because so much has been accomplished, we have expected a great deal more than has been achieved. It seems as though almost every day a new drug or surgical technique is reported in the public press and the implication has gradually become accepted that there are no bounds to what we may hope to accomplish by this approach. We have verged on believing that we might not only cure all the ills of the flesh we are subject to, but indeed all the pains and problems that are a part of the human condition.

As more and more problems—mental and spiritual as well as physical—were taken over by the medical profession as belonging to their province, our definition of *health* became far larger than "absence of disease." We have begun to expect the physician not only to prevent and cure our disease, but also to make us healthy. By this we mean, in a vague and undefined way, full of zest, gusto, and the enjoyment of life. These, however, are goals that the physician is not trained to help us attain. Health is a state of being in which our physical, mental, and spiritual needs are being fulfilled and expressed in a way unique to ourselves. Healthy, we can, if we try hard enough, make an artistic creation out of our entire lives, a sort of symphony, in which first one theme and then another takes predominance. It is the task of the physician to make this state achievable by helping us to cure our physical ills. It is not his task, nor within his training, to do more than this.

In holistic health centers physicians and practitioners of the adjunctive modalities such as nutrition and acupuncture are learning to work together. Within this process some individuals are learning to work with the whole patient and are developing into health specialists. In other areas such as the "liaison psychiatry" now found in many hospitals, a holistic health attitude is being developed and experimented with. Many individual physicians in their everyday work have gone far beyond the narrow bounds of their medical school training and are viewing and responding to their patients on many levels of existence.

Although many people are experimenting with this method, we have not yet really begun to train the kind of specialist who can help us achieve health. There are some wise physicians trying to combine the roles of disease specialist and health specialist. Indeed, it would be ideal if they could be combined in one person. Since the present training for the disease specialist is so extensive, however, and since there are definite personality and training requirements for the health specialist, it is probable that in the foreseeable future separate persons usually will have to fill the roles.

We have just begun to train health specialists. We can say a good deal about them, what they will have to do, the kind of personality they will need, what kind of training they will require, and how they can work closely with the disease specialist. Until we develop this field much further, however, each of us will have to function as his own health specialist.

The health specialist will work according to the basic assumptions that have emerged from the newly developing field of holistic medicine. There are four assumptions:

1. The individual person exists on many levels. These include the physical, the emotional, the mental, and the spiritual. All of them are equally important in achieving health. None is "more real" than any other. One may choose to concentrate on a single aspect first with a particular patient, but all must be taken into account.
2. The patient has self-healing and self-repair systems and they must be regarded as crucial in the prevention and cure of disease.
3. The patient must be actively and knowledgeably involved in his own treatment and in designing a program to work toward health.
4. Each person is a unique individual and must be met and responded to as such.

Holistic medicine is a set of concepts, not a precise set of techniques. There are a very large number of adjunctive modalities available today, ranging from nutrition to meditation, and they include a wide variety of specific techniques. Very often the practitioners and teachers of these modalities believe and claim that they are involved in a "holistic medicine" approach, but have little idea of what that is in actuality. If they claim, as they sometimes do, that their way is the only way to health and that all you need to do to achieve health is to eat what they suggest or meditate in their style or have your muscles aligned according to their principles, they are certainly not followers of the cardinal principles of holistic medicine. It is necessary to have a comprehensive and enthusiastic acceptance of all four of the principles, not just an involvement with a modality of treatment that is not accepted by mainline medicine.

Since a basic tenet of this approach is that *all* levels of the person are equally important, there are no such things as "alternative modalities." There are only "adjunctive modalities," approaches that are used *in addition* to an orthodox medical approach in the treatment of disease. If no disease is present, they may be used as means for self-development. Many of them can be used to great benefit. Any intelligent program for our own health, however, must follow certain rules. It must be uniquely designed for the individual and not mass produced. It must involve the person concerned as an active and knowledgeable participant. It must be seen as part of the answer to our problems of growth and being, not *the* answer. There are also ways of evaluating practitioners of the adjunctive modalities, including their ability to work with other specialists (such as mainline physicians) in helping the person prevent and cure disease and work toward health.

With the growth of the modern hospital to its present size and complexity, and the probability that each of us, or someone we are very close to, will spend some time in one eventually, it is important that we know how to behave so as to receive the maximum benefit from our stay. To do this requires certain preparation. We must be aware that a hospital is a business selling tests and medical procedures. If we are in a stressful situation such as that caused by certain illnesses, surgical procedures, or tests, we need to have a strong advocate who will be with us as much as possible and who will be able to act strongly in our behalf. The pressures in the modern hospital to relinquish one's adult status and behave as a helpless and "good" child are very strong and must be resisted if we are to do as well as possible while we are there.

The importance of taking control of one's own destiny in matters of disease and of health is a central idea of the emerging field of holistic medicine. If one is willing to take responsibility in this way, one can get the best from both mainline medicine and the adjunctive modalities. One can increase resistance to disease, receive the greatest possible benefits from medical treatment if and when it is needed, and can move toward a state of health that will bring the best and richest life possible.

A great medical researcher of the mid-nineteenth century, Rudolf Virchow, regarded disease as "life under changed conditions" and concluded that the physician had to concern himself with the total environment of human beings, and therefore must also take part in political action.

To give a simple example: If malnutrition is so often the foster parent of infection, where does the physician's task stop? We are becoming aware that both the disease specialist and the health specialist are going to have to take an active role in social affairs. The interaction of the social and biological realms is seen most clearly in the world's foremost cause of death, the diarrhea-pneumonia syndrome that accounts for the majority of the huge infant mortality rate in underdeveloped countries. It is not caused by any specific virus or bacterium, but results from the overall pattern of heredity, nutrition, and sanitation factors.

Adlai Stevenson wrote:

We all travel together, passengers on a little spaceship, dependent on its vulnerable supplies of air and soil, all committed for our safety to its security and peace, preserved from annihilation only by the care, the work, and I will say the love we give our fragile craft.

Although I have concerned myself primarily with the issues of disease and health, the major underlying concern has to do with nothing more or less than mankind's survival on earth!

Far beyond the questions of what may or may not happen in a doctor's office, or in a hospital operating room, or the way in which we learn to prevent illness in ourselves or participate in the healing process, is the question of whether or not our planet will remain habitable.

The real health-illness issue is this: Can human beings stop worshiping technology in time? Can they begin to use technology in terms of human values and stop seeing it as a value in itself? The mathematician Norbert Wiener has suggested an Eleventh Commandment for the twentieth century—"Render unto man that which belongs to man and unto computers that which belongs to computers." And most urgent of all: Can we stop fouling our own nest? It makes no difference what medical professionals or health professionals can or cannot do, if we have no clean water to drink, if our food is poisoned by chemicals in the soil, if we so destroy the balance in nature that human life becomes insupportable.

These awful things need not happen—but time is running out. Each of us not only must take care of his own life, but must express active concern for the lives of all human beings.

Notes

Page   CHAPTER 1: THE PRESENT SITUATION IN
          MEDICINE

9   "That any sane nation . . .": George Bernard Shaw, Preface to
          The Doctor's Dilemma.

9   "Nothing has changed . . .": Lewis Thomas, "On the Science
          and Technology of Medicine," in John H. Knowles, ed., *Doing
          Better and Feeling Worse* (New York: W. W. Norton, 1977),
          p. 43.

10   "No one takes . . .": Ibid.

10   In spite of: Ibid., p. 35.

11   "A typical case . . .": Ibid., p. 37.

14   "In our society . . .": Eric J. Cassell, *The Healer's Art* (Philadel-
          phia and New York: Lippincott, 1976), p. 129.

15   Birds, for example: Kenneth Walker, *Patients and Doctors*
          (Harmondsworth, Middlesex: Penguin, 1957), p. 14.

16   C. W. Hufeland: quoted in S. Peller, "Mortality Past and Pres-
          ent," *Population Studies*, Vol. 1, No. 4, March, 1948, p. 406.

17–18   The medicalization of American Society: Renée C. Fox, "The
          Medicalization and Demedicalization of American Society," in
          John H. Knowles, ed., *Doing Better and Feeling Worse* (New
          York: W. W. Norton, 1977).

20   Drugs and alcohol: Martin R. Lipp, *Respectful Treatment* (Ha-
          gerstown, Md.: Medical Dept., Harper and Row, 1977), p. 206.

22   In one experiment: D. L. Rosenhan, "On Being Sane in Insane
          Places," *Science*, 179 (1973), pp. 250–58.

22   An experiment with: Richard Rennecker, personal communica-
          tion (1975).

23   "In more than . . .": Thomas Szasz, *The Manufacture of Mad-
          ness* (New York: Delta, 1970), p. 55.

23   With our increased: Herbert R. Kohl, *The Age of Complexity*
          (New York: New American Library, 1965).

28   One patient with: Victor Hive, *Last Letter to the Pebble People*
          (Miami: St. Aldens in the Woods, 1977).

29   "The present trend . . .": Alexis Carrel, *Man, the Unknown*
          (London: Hamish Hamilton, 1935), p. 29.

30   "Instead of resembling . . .": Ibid., p. 392.
31   "The dominant model . . .": George L. Engel, "The Need for a
          New Medical Model: A Challenge for Biomedicine," *Science*,
          196 (1977), pp. 129–136, p. 130.
31   ". . . a genuine discrepancy . . .": Ibid., p. 135.
33   "I was once . . .": Sidney M. Jourard, *The Transparent Self*
          (Princeton, N.J.: Van Nostrand Reinhold, 1964).
34   "Medicine's crisis stems . . .": George L. Engel, "The Need for a
          New Medical Model: A Challenge for Biomedicine," *Science*
          196 (1977), p. 129.
34   "A seventy-eight-year-old man . . .": Nancy L. Caroline, "Dying
          in Academe," in Peretz, et al., eds., *Death and Grief: Selected
          Readings for Medical Students* (New York: Health Science
          Publ. Corp., 1977), pp. 17–20.
35   ". . . it makes no sense . . .": Martin R. Lipp, *Respectful Treat-
          ment* (Hagerstown, Md.: Medical Dept., Harper and Row,
          1977), p. 1.
36   "All honour to those . . .": *Lancet* 1 (1964), p. 76.
37   "A program to improve . . .": John H. Knowles, "The Responsi-
          bility of the Individual," in John H. Knowles, ed., *Doing Better
          and Feeling Worse* (New York: W. W. Norton, 1977), p. 77.
37   Sociology of medicine: Amasa B. Ford, *Urban Health in Amer-
          ica* (New York: Oxford University Press, 1970), p. ix.
38–39   "A manifestation of . . .": Robert Swearingen, *Journal of Holis-
          tic Health* 5 (1980), pp. 44–45.

Page   CHAPTER 2: THE MECHANIC AND THE GAR-
          DENER: TWO APPROACHES TO DISEASE AND
          HEALTH
44   Eisenbud's First Theorem: An aphorism coined some years ago
          by the psychoanalyst Jules Eisenbud.
46   "Galen has already . . .": Maimonides, *The Preservation of
          Youth*, trans. Hirsch L. Gordon (New York: Philosophical Li-
          brary, 1958), p. 38.
47   Thus, from his viewpoint: K. M. Yost, "Sydenham's Philosophy
          of Science," *Osiris* 9 (1950), pp. 84–105. One Eastern system—
          Ayurvedic or Tibetan medicine—developed in close parallel to
          the Theory of Humors of Galenic medicine. The Ayurvedic sys-
          tem has three humors—mucus, wind, and fire—instead of the
          Western four. It also sees disease as resulting from the excess
          of humors (*doshas*) and its effect on the body. Because of the
          lack of a scientific revolution in the East, they never made

much progress beyond this, and are still using what we would call today a medieval viewpoint in medicine.

47   The comments they made: Marie Boas, *The Scientific Renaissance, 1450–1630* (New York: Harper Torchbooks, 1962), p. 160.

48   "Descartes's ... description": Ivan Illich, *Medical Nemesis* (New York: Bantam, 1977), p. 156. Voltaire wrote: "The art of medicine consists of amusing the patient while nature heals the disease": quoted in Irving Oyle, *The New American Medicine Show* (Santa Cruz: Unit Press, 1979), p. 33.

48   Against the rising tide: Charles E. Raven, *Science, Medicine and Morals* (New York: Harper & Bros., 1959), p. 29.

49   On one side: Richard H. Shryock, *Medical Licensing in America, 1650–1965* (Baltimore: Johns Hopkins Press, 1967).

49–50 "The Constitution of this ...": quoted as epigraph in Brian Inglis, *The Case for Unorthodox Medicine* (New York: G. P. Putnam's Sons, 1967).

51   "... that where the ...": Ibid., p. 8.

53–54 "Although occasionally ...": Ibid., p. 48.

55   "... The partnership ...": Kenneth Walker, *Patients and Doctors* (Harmondsworth, Middlesex: Penguin, 1957), pp. 23–24.

56   When we read: Geoffrey Marks and William K. Beatty, *Epidemics* (New York: Scribner's, 1976), pp. 21ff.

56   "During these times ...": Procopius, trans. H. B. Dewing (London: Heinemann, 1914), pp. 451ff.

57   "Illnesses hover constantly ...": quoted in Dennis Jaffee, *Healing From Within* (New York: Knopf, 1980), p. 15.

57   The *context* of disease: René Dubos, *Mirage of Health* (New York: Harper and Row, 1979), p. 105.

57   Thirty-five percent died: Gotthard Booth, *The Cancer Epidemic: Shadow of the Conquest of Nature* (New York: E. Mellen Press, 1979), p. 19.

58   Less than 2 percent: Richard Doll, "Cancer: The Possibilities," *British Medical Journal*, 1 (1965), p. 471.

59   Widowers have a: Arthur S. Kraus and Abraham Lilienfeld, "Some Epidemiologic Aspects of the High Mortality Rate in the Young Widowed Group," *Journal of Chronic Diseases*, 10 (3), (1959), pp. 207–217.

59   "In an industrial ...": Eric J. Cassell, "Psychosocial Processes and 'Stress': Theoretical Formulations," in Charles A. Garfield, ed., *Stress and Survival* (St. Louis: C. V. Mosby Co., 1979), p. 48.

59   "... the microbial diseases ...": René Dubos, *Mirage of Health*
            (New York: Harper and Row, 1979), p. 104.
59–60   "Alteration of the ...": Eric J. Cassell, "Psychosocial Processes
            and 'Stress': Theoretical Formulations," in Charles A. Garfield
            ed., *Stress and Survival* (St. Louis: C. V. Mosby Co., 1979),
            p. 47.
60   "... the will to live ...": Norman Cousins, "Anatomy of an Ill-
            ness," in Garfield, p. 171.
60   "A medicine's value ...": Kenneth Walker, *Patients and Doc-
            tors* (Harmondsworth, Middlesex: Penguin, 1957), p. 96.
60–61   "The most common ...": Francis W. Peabody, "The Care of the
            Patient," *Journal of the American Medical Association*, 88
            (1927), p. 877.
61   "... let me speak ...": Iris Origo, *The Merchant of Prato* (New
            York: Knopf, 1957).
64   Jon Garfield has: Jon Garfield, "Social Stress and Medical Ideol-
            ogy," in Charles A. Garfield, ed., *Stress and Survival* (St. Louis:
            C. V. Mosby Co., 1979), p. 33
65   Typical of: Martin R. Lipp,/*Respectful Treatment* (Hagerstown,
            Md.: Medical Dept., Harper and Row, 1977).
65–66   "Anyone who has ...": quoted by Charles A. Garfield, ed.,
            Stress and Survival (St. Louis: C. V. Mosby Co., 1979).
66–67   "When we pass ...": Kenneth Walker, *Patients and Doctors*
            (Harmondsworth, Middlesex: Penguin, 1951), p. 96.
68–69   "Looking back at ...": Lewis Thomas, "The Right Track," *East-
            ern Review* (September 1980), pp. 43ff.

Page   CHAPTER 3: THE SCIENTIFIC REVOLUTION OF
            THE TWENTIETH CENTURY
77   "Half a century ...": N. Rashevsky, "Is the concept of the or-
            ganism as a machine a useful one?" in P. S. Frank, ed., *The
            Validation of Scientific Theories* (Boston: Beacon Press,
            1954).
77   "... the popular metaphysic ...": S. Langer, "On Cassirer's
            Theory of Language and Myth," in Paul Schilpp, *The Philos-
            ophy of Ernst Cassirer* (Evanston, Ill.: Library of Living Philos-
            ophies, 1977), p. 381.
78   This is not: Albert Einstein and Leopold Infeld, *The Evolution
            of Physics* (New York: Simon and Schuster, 1965); Henry Mar-
            genau, *The Nature of Physical Reality* (New York: McGraw-
            Hill, 1950); Sir Arthur Eddington, *The Nature of the Physical
            World* (New York: Macmillan, 1931).

78   "Each system of . . .": Alexis Carrel, *Man, the Unknown* (London: Hamish Hamilton, 1935), p. 43.

Page   CHAPTER 4: THE APPLICATION OF THE NEW
         SCIENTIFIC REVOLUTION TO MEDICINE
84   ". . . health is not . . .": M. C. Todd, "The Need for a New Health Program," in Edward Bauman, A. Brint, L. Piper, and P. Wright, eds., *The Holistic Health Handbook* (Berkeley, Calif.: And/Or Press, 1978), p. 26.
86   "A 'thing' is . . .": Edward B. Titchener, *An Outline of Psychology* (New York: Macmillan, 1886), p. 5.
88   "These are Abraham Maslow's": Abraham H. Maslow, *Toward a Psychology of Being* (New York: Van Nostrand Reinhold, 1962).
91–92   "We have acquired . . .": René Dubos, *So Human an Animal* (New York: Scribner's, 1968), p. xi.

Page   CHAPTER 5: THE HEALTH SPECIALIST
95   "It is hardly conceivable . . .": Franz Alexander, "Fundamental Concepts of Psychosomatic Research," *Psychosomatic Medicine* V (1943), p. 206.
96   The importance of context: Levy Bruhl, *La Mentalité Primitif* (Paris, 1933).
97   Excellent reviews: Brian Inglis, *The Case for Unorthodox Healing* (New York: G. P. Putnam's Sons, 1969).
97   Excellent reviews of: Jerome Frank, *Persuasion And Healing* (Baltimore: Johns Hopkins Press, 1961).
97–99   "In the summer of 1962 . . .": Brian Inglis, *The Case for Unorthodox Medicine* (New York: G. P. Putnam's Sons, 1967), pp. 43–44.
100   "There is no valid . . .": William James, quoted in Kurt Goldstein, *Human Nature* (Cambridge: Harvard University Press, 1951), p. 9.
101   "Placed on this . . .": Alexander Pope, *Essay on Man*, Epistle II, 1. 3–18.
102   ". . . solving problems . . .": René Dubos, *Mirage of Health* (New York: Harper and Row, 1979), p. 26.
102   "When a student . . .": Kurt Goldstein, *Human Nature* (Cambridge: Harvard University Press, 1951), p. 9.
103   As the philosopher: Ibid., p. 113.
103–04 "The disadvantages of . . .": Kenneth Walker, *Patients and Doctors* (Harmondsworth, Middlesex: Penguin, 1957), p. 96.

104   "... We are far more ...": Ibid., p. 32.

106   "The real guru ...": Pin Vilayet Khan, quoted from a lecture given in New York City, March 17, 1977.

107   "Man masters nature ...": Jacob Bronowski, *Science and Human Values* (New York: Harper and Row, 1965), p. 10.

108   The patient essentially: Thomas Szasz and Marc H. Hollander, "A Contribution to the Philosophy of Medicine," A.M.A. *Archives of Internal Medicine* XCVII (1956), pp. 585–92.

108   "The patient has to ...": Marvin Meilus, personal communication (1979).

110   Doing so shows respect: Editorial, *Lancet* (1948), p. 760, quoted in Martin R. Lipp, *Respectful Treatment* (New York: Harper and Row, 1977), p. 61.

110   "Find your own ...": Hans Selye, "Stress without Distress," in Charles A. Garfield, ed., *Stress and Survival* (St. Louis: C. V. Mosby Co., 1979), p. 13.

111   "It is impossible ...": Martin Buber, *The Way of Man* (Secaucus, N.J.: Citadel Press, 1973), pp. 9ff.

114   "... any response ...": Florence Miale, personal communication (1970).

118   "... there is a real ...": Virginia Veach, personal communication (1980).

119   "God exercises ...": St. Thomas Aquinas, *Summa contra gentiles*, Book 3, chapter 122.

119   "The more perfect ...": Maimonides, *The Preservation of Youth* (New York: Philosophical Library, 1958), p. 79.

121   "Self-actualization ...": Abraham H. Maslow, *Toward a Psychology of Being* (New York: Van Nostrand Reinhold, 1962), p. 102.

121   "The secret of ...": Francis W. Peabody, "The Care of the Patient," *Journal of the American Medical Association* 88 (1927), p. 882.

124   "I said to the almond ...": Nikos Kazantzakis, *Report to Greco* (New York: Bantam, 1965), p. 2.

Page   CHAPTER   6:   WORKING   FOR   YOUR   OWN HEALTH: HOW TO BE YOUR OWN HEALTH SPECIALIST

125   "The equal and cooperative ...": quoted in "Raven," *Science, Medicine and Morals* (New York: Harper & Bros., 1959), p. 26.

125–26 "Even if present ...": Eric J. Cassell, *The Healer's Art* (Philadelphia and New York: Lippincott, 1976), p. 75.

126   "Cancer is no . . .": quoted in G. Booth, *The Cancer Epidemic: Shadow of the Conquest of Nature* (New York: E. Mellen Press, 1979), p. 20.

126   Hans Selye: Hans Selye, in a lecture, "Cancer Dialogue, 80" (New York, 1980).

126   The first artificial: S. J. Reiser, "Therapeutic Choice and Moral Doubt in a Technological Age," in John H. Knowles, *Doing Better and Feeling Worse* (New York: W. W. Norton, 1977), pp. 47–56, p. 53.

127   "The majority of doctors . . .": H. P. Drietsch, "Introduction: The Social Organization of Health," in H. P. Drietsch, ed., *The Social Organization of Health* (New York: Macmillan, 1971), p. 7.

133   "The practice of medicine . . .": Sir William Osler, *The Master Word in Medicine* (Baltimore: John Murphy, 1903), p. 29.

137   The writer and poet: May Sarton, *Mrs. Stevens Hears the Mermaids Singing* (New York: W. W. Norton, 1975), p. 181.

138   ". . . the most compelling . . .": René Dubos, *Mirage of Health* (New York: Harper and Row, 1979), p. 26.

138   "Every age but . . .": Abraham H. Maslow, *Toward a Psychology of Being* (New York: Van Nostrand Reinhold, 1962), p. 4.

139   When individuals with: Lawrence LeShan, *You Can Fight for Your Life: Emotional Factors in the Treatment of Cancer* (New York: Evans, 1979).

140   In his autobiography: Nikos Kazantzakis, *Report to Greco* (New York: Bantam, 1965), p. 13.

Special resources for information on the adjunctive modalities of treatment: Ann Hill, ed., *The Visual Encyclopedia of Unconventional Medicine* (New York: Crown Publishers, 1979). Edward Bauman, A. Brint, L. Piper, and P. Wright, eds., *The Holistic Health Handbook* (Berkeley: And/Or Press, 1978). Leslie J. Kaslof, *Wholistic Dimensions in Healing: a Resource Guide* (Garden City, N.Y.: Doubleday, 1978). These books survey the entire field of adjunctive modalities and describe each of them. They also refer to specialized books on each specific modality for further reading.

Page   **CHAPTER 7: THE PRACTICE OF HOLISTIC MEDICINE: CASE HISTORIES AND DEMONSTRATIONS OF THE METHOD**

151   ". . . learning to use . . .": Ilana Rubenfeld, personal communication (1980).

153   It was *this*: Western mysticism in particular has always been (as *The Cloud of Unknowing*, a medieval manuscript, put it)

"listy"—the opposite of "listless"—active and involved in the world. St. John of the Cross wrote in his *Ascent of Mount Carmel*: "How much more in God's sight is one act of the will performed in charity than are all the visions and communications they may receive from heaven."

155   Originated by Carl Simonton: Carl Simonton, S. Simonton and J. Creighton, *Getting Well Again* (Los Angeles: J. P. Tancher, 1978).

155–56   "During psychotherapy": The psychotherapy method is described in Lawrence LeShan, *You Can Fight for Your Life* (New York: Evans, 1980).

159   Working regularly with: For further descriptions of this and other meditation forms and their effects, see, Lawrence LeShan, *How to Meditate* (New York: Bantam, 1975); Claudio Naranjo and R. Ornstein, *The Psychology of Meditation* (New York: Viking, 1971); and Evelyn Underhill, *Practical Mysticism* (London: S. M. Dent, 1914).

164   "The point being . . .": Emanuel Cheraskin, "Nutrition: A Basis for Health," *Journal of Holistic Health* 5 (1980), pp. 49–55, p. 53.

169   "The rule accepted . . .": quoted in George Vithoulkas, "Homeopathy," in Bauman, et al., *The Holistic Health Handbook* (Berkeley: And/Or Press, 1978), p. 88.

Page   **CHAPTER 8: HOW TO SURVIVE IN A HOSPITAL**
183   "How many heroic . . .": René Dubos, *Mirage of Health* (New York: Harper and Row, 1979), p. 62.

187   "From that moment . . .": Edgar N. Jackson, *Coping with the Crises of Your Life* (New York: Hawthorne Books, 1974), p. 15.

188   "It has often been said . . .": quoted in Irving Oyle, *The New American Medicine Show* (Santa Cruz: Unity Press, 1979), p. 25.

191   Once you have: Some of the following comments on necessary information are a paraphrase of: Francis V. Chisari, Robert M. Nakamura, and Lorena Thorup, *The Consumer's Guide to Health Care* (Boston: Little Brown, 1970), p. 5.

191   Unless there is a coordinating: Martin R. Lipp, *Respectful Treatment* (Hagerstown, Md.: Medical Dept., Harper and Row, 1977), p. 2.

192   Between 1967 and 1972: George L. Engel, "The Need for a New Medical Model: A Challenge for Biomedicine," *Science* 196 (1977), p. 135.

192–93 "Some medical students . . .": Eric J. Cassell, *The Healer's Art* (Philadelphia and New York: Lippincott, 1976), p. 106.

193   One study showed: Herbert Benson, *The Mind/Body Effect* (New York: Berkeley Books, 1980), p. 77.

196   In 1972: Martin R. Lipp, *Respectful Treatment* (Hagerstown, Md.: Medical Dept., Harper and Row, 1977), p. 64.

197   Incidentally, the small number: Ibid., p. 48.

198   In 1934: Harry Bakwin, "Pseudodoxia Pediatrica," *New England Journal of Medicine* CCXXII (1945), pp. 691–697.

207   A great medical researcher: René Dubos, *Mirage of Health* (New York: Harper and Row, 1979), p. 110.

207   "We all travel . . .": Adlai E. Stevenson, Talk at United Nations Economic and Social Council, Geneva, July 9, 1965. Quoted in René Dubos, *So Human an Animal*, p. 261.